FOR EVERYONE
WHO SEEKS BETTER HEALTH AND HEALTH CARE

Do what you can, where you are, with what you have.

Theodore Roosevelt

CONTENTS

PREFACE

My life has been saved by doctors and hospitals on at least three occasions: first, before I was born, when my mother went into labor two months early; second, in my teens, when I nearly stopped breathing as a result of a massive allergic reaction; and third, in my thirties, when I needed brain surgery.

I have a profound appreciation for the intelligence, training, experience, and dedication of everyone who contributes to terrific outcomes in health care. The list includes doctors, nurses, pharmacists, hospital administrators, researchers who come up with the drugs and devices used to save lives, and millions of others without whom health care would simply grind to a halt.

The health care system does a wonderful job of describing its great successes. For example, billboards advertising miracles in treating heart attacks and cancer are common sights. The health care system doesn't need any help promoting its benefits.

But that's only half of the story. *Killer Cure* highlights the other half. Health care in the United States has massive shortcomings which can entirely cancel out the great benefits that it can deliver.

My intentions in writing *Killer Cure* are twofold. The first is to help you, the reader, recognize and understand the gaps that put you at risk when you deal with the health care system. It is only with this knowledge that you have a chance to reduce your risk.

The second intention is to offer you a new perspective that can enable you to think very differently about your health, about your health care, and about how you interact with the health care system. My goal is to improve the odds that health care will *increase* rather than *decrease* your ability to lead the life you want.

People who have heard me speak about this perspective have later told me that it has permanently changed how they think and act in the realm of health care. Many of them have said things like, "Everybody needs to hear this! When are you going to write a book?" I wrote *Killer Cure* in response.

A number of the stories in *Killer Cure* that describe gaps in care are drawn from my own experience. Many of them unfolded over many months. Because I kept detailed records of my care, it was possible to look back afterwards and identify what went wrong at various points along the way.

These stories illustrate that interactions with the health care system can be filled with life-diminishing and even life-threatening challenges — even for people who don't have any serious chronic diseases. I include my own stories not because they are so unusual, but precisely because, at their core, they are not. I hope that in doing so, I give voice to your experience and that of your family and friends.

It's important to note that when the shortcomings in health care involve doctors as the main actors, their mental or emotional state almost never includes malice or ill will. Virtually every health care professional, by all accounts, arrives at work every day with good intentions.

The worst that can be said is that they may not recognize the unintended consequences of their assumptions and of their actions. One might say that perhaps they have a blind spot, or possibly a kind of tunnel vision. They certainly don't mean to hurt anyone.

There is a light at the end of the tunnel. Change is coming. The only question is, when will it arrive? I wrote *Killer Cure* both to help hasten its coming and to assist you until it does.

The endnotes are extensive. The reason is that much of the picture painted about "the other half" of what happens in health care — the part that doesn't make it onto billboards — is so shocking that I imagine you may want to be able to refer to the research and references that underlie it. Besides providing references, the endnotes offer additional quotations, analyses, and explanations.

A word about terminology: throughout the book, I refer to "health care" or "the health care system" as if it were an organized entity that is capable of making decisions and taking action. Most experts would say that health care typically is not that tidy — it is usually fragmented and uncoordinated. That assessment is entirely accurate.

I use the terms "health care" and "health care system" simply as shorthand to avoid having to say, "the doctors, nurses, hospital administrators, pharmacists, insurance companies, lawmakers, researchers, drug and device manufacturers, aides, clerks, and so forth" every time I refer to the people and organizations that play a role in the delivery of care.

At the end of *Killer Cure* is a Readers' Discussion Guide. It is offered to aid you in thinking about and discussing both the book and your own experiences with health care.

I wish you all the best.

CHAPTER ONE

It's Not the Health Care System You Think It Is; or, "Pay no attention to the man behind the curtain."

Health care is dangerous to your health. Doctors mean well. However, health care gone wrong kills more Americans every week *than were killed in the first six years of the war in Iraq. You can learn what the problems are so that you can reap the benefits of health care while avoiding tragic mishaps.*

Broken Heart

Bob was born with four holes in his heart. One of them was larger than his aorta. Experts deemed it the most severe and complicated case they had ever seen. His doctors didn't tell his parents, Shannon and Jeff, that it was almost guaranteed that their baby would die.

But Bob deteriorated before their eyes. He started turning blue when feeding, and soon refused to eat at all — sucking was too much work for his weakened heart. A feeding tube was inserted, and night after night Jeff and Shannon set the alarm to wake up every three hours to feed him. Each feeding took an hour, and Bob vomited up most of what he took in.

His doctors wanted him to gain weight before they considered surgery, which was almost certain to be futile anyway. But even with the feeding tube, he barely held his ground. At three months, he weighed little more than he had at birth.

At one point he was in the hospital for a week straight. Shannon and Jeff were exhausted, but one of them was with the baby 24 hours a day. Jeff's employer was very understanding, but there were still times when he needed to go to work. As a result Shannon covered the day shift and many of the evening and night shifts.

The nurses kept telling her that she didn't have to be there all the time. They encouraged her to go home and rest. She refused, scarcely leaving her baby's side. She explained,

"He was just lying in a crib in a room. They wouldn't necessarily hear him cry. If he needed something, it's not like he could press the call button."

At one point in the grueling ordeal, Shannon looked up to see a nurse enter the room with a syringe full of medicine to inject into Bob's IV. Shannon had noticed that one of his drugs had a cloudy appearance, and one was clear. One had a high dose, and one a low dose.

Startled by what she saw in the syringe, she blurted out, "That's three times what he usually gets!" It was just seconds before the nurse would plunge the needle into the baby's IV. The nurse looked at her quizzically and then left the room. She returned a moment later, visibly shaken.

Bob was supposed to get a high dose of a drug to eliminate excess fluid from his system, and a low dose of a drug to slow his heart rate so that his heart didn't have to work so hard. The nurse had reversed the doses of the two drugs.

She had nearly injected a massive overdose of the heart-slowing drug into his IV. It would have killed him on the spot. Bob's life was saved only because Shannon wasn't in the bathroom or getting a cup of coffee when the nurse showed up.

A week or so later, Shannon was able to get Bob in to see a surgeon who was reputed to be the best in the country for pediatric heart problems. He warned her that the outcome was uncertain; the position of the holes would make it very difficult to operate. But he thought he might be able to save her son.

Having struggled his entire life — from Easter to the Fourth of July — Bob now lay in one of the best pediatric hospitals in the country, awaiting open heart surgery. Kept alive only by potent drugs, he was perhaps a week from death. He slept almost all the time now; just being awake was too much effort.

Doctor after doctor examined him. Shannon was grateful and encouraged; they were all so attentive to her tiny son. She didn't find out until later that they were doctors in training who were eager to see this critically ill infant because his case was so unusual and extreme that it would be a miracle if he survived.

The day of surgery arrived. Repairing multiple hard-to-reach holes in an organ about the size of a walnut, the extraordinarily gifted surgeon turned in an astonishing performance, and Bob survived the surgery.

As a result, Jeff and Shannon started to hope that their desperately ill baby might have a shot at a normal life, a chance to see other Easters and other Fourths of July, a chance to see Halloween and Thanksgiving and Christmas.

Bob's care is a microcosm of health care in America: catastrophic failures in the basics and incredible miracles in the dramatic, all mixed together. In his case, the miracles won out: years after death-defying surgery, Bob is an intelligent, active, cheerful human being.

Not everyone is so lucky.

Russian Roulette

In the U.S., over 12,000 people die *every week* from health care gone awry.[1] Said another way, that's about 624,000 deaths a year.

These aren't people who die because of the illness or injury that brings them to the doctor. These are people who die because of the care they receive once they get there.[2] In fact, you stand a one-in-four chance that your death will be *caused* by medical care.[3]

Russian roulette offers better odds.

It's not the health care system you think it is. There is no Wizard of Oz in health care — all-seeing, all-knowing, all-powerful — who will make you better in all but the gravest cases when you are ill. Health care providers would understandably like you to have confidence in the care they give, so there's a tendency for them to say, "Pay no attention to the man behind the curtain," as the Wizard of Oz did when his hiding place was exposed and he was discovered to be a mere mortal.

A few facts might surprise you:

- The U.S. ranks 50th in the world in life expectancy. Americans live shorter lives than Bosnians and not much longer than Albanians.[4]
- The U.S. ranks 46th in the world in infant survival rates. That's behind Cuba and just a little ahead of Croatia.[5] As Nicholas Kristof wrote in the *New York Times*, "If the U.S. had an infant mortality rate as good as Cuba's, we would save an additional 2,212 American babies a year."[6]
- The World Health Organization ranks the U.S. health care system overall 37th in the world. That's right after Costa Rica and just before Slovenia.[7]

If this picture is news to you, you might find it hard to believe. You might even be outraged — not at these statistics, but that someone would dare to suggest that our health care system isn't the best in the world. You might be wondering what the catch is, the statistical gimmick, the game being played with the numbers.

There isn't one.

Lacerated Uterus

Consider what can — and too often does — go wrong with the basics. The causes of those 12,000 deaths each week fall into four categories:

- medical errors in hospitals
- infections transmitted to patients in hospitals
- blood clots in hospitals
- adverse drug events

Medical errors include everything from operating on the wrong patient to transfusing someone with the wrong blood type. These aren't judgment calls. These aren't situations in which there are two different opinions about the best course of treatment. These are just mistakes.

About 200,000 people die each year in this country due to medical error,[8] and one study suggested that about 87% of those deaths are preventable.[9] What are some of the main types of medical errors?

- use of outmoded tests or treatment
- error in performing an operation or a test
- failure to act when an abnormal test result shows that prompt action is needed
- failure of communication
- equipment failure[10]

Lauren's story provides a non-fatal example of medical errors. A few months after Lauren and her husband got married, they were thrilled to discover that she was pregnant. She miscarried, though, and six months later got pregnant again. She miscarried again.

Each of the miscarriages required a D&C (dilation and curettage), a simple outpatient procedure. However, the second D&C wasn't done quite right — the first medical error in this situation — and she had to return to the hospital six weeks later for a repeat D&C.

She awoke from the anesthesia to find the doctor leaning over her, explaining that he had perforated Lauren's uterus in two places in the course of doing the repeat D&C. This is the second medical error (or second and third, depending on how one counts). The surgeon attempted to repair the lacerations with minimally invasive procedures, but in the end had to make a large incision in Lauren's abdomen.

Even non-fatal medical errors have consequences. In Lauren's case, the first error led to another hospital stay. The second/third error(s) meant that instead of being in and out of the hospital in a few hours, she spent several days there. Then she was not permitted to drive for two weeks, and was permitted to return to the office only part-time for four weeks. Other limitations on heavy lifting, exercise, and other activities were in place for six weeks.

Was the fact that she was never able to get pregnant after that related to the lacerations and repairs? Lauren and her husband will never know.

The medical errors in that experience are considered minor.

Invisible Enemy

Separate from the incidence of medical errors is the fact that about 1.7 million people each year pick up infections while in the hospital, and 99,000 die as a result.[11] These are not old people who are so frail and sick that they are going to die anyway. These are people who check in to the hospital to have, say, elective knee surgery. They check out via the morgue.

In 1847 an Austrian-Hungarian obstetrician, Ignaz Semmelweis, discovered that mortality in hospitals could be cut dramatically if people washed their hands and instruments before working on patients. At the time, the mortality rate for women giving birth was 10-35%.

The death rates were much higher on wards serviced by doctors than on those serviced by midwives. It turned out that the doctors were coming to the wards straight from performing autopsies, without having washed their hands.[12]

Doctors were outraged at the suggestion that they were causing deaths — after all, they were the good guys — and believed that it was simply inevitable that many women would die in childbirth.

Hospital infections are not inevitable.[13] Hospitals in other countries, and some in the U.S., have dramatically reduced the percent of patients who get them.[14]

How are infections typically transmitted in hospitals today? One study showed that when doctors and nurses lean over patients, their clothing picks up bacteria 65% of the time — easily transferred to the next patient.[15] One outbreak of infection studied was apparently the result of nursing assistants emptying bedpans and delivering meals in the same clothes.[16]

However, the main method of transmission is by care providers who don't wash their hands.[17] In fact, only about a third of hospital workers routinely wash their hands before touching patients.[18] Doctors are not exempt: fewer than half wash their hands "if they think no one is watching."[19]

Today more people die from hospital-acquired infections than die from breast cancer (41,000/year)[20] and automobile accidents (45,000/year)[21] put together. Said another way, hand washing might save twice as many lives as would a miracle cure that completely eliminated breast cancer.

It is disheartening to realize that an indisputable discovery made 160 years ago, which could readily save nearly a million lives a decade, has yet to be routinely reflected in practice.

Blood Clots

Blood clots that form in the veins and then break off and travel to the lungs cause about 200,000 deaths after surgery or hospitalization for other treatment.[22]

These are considered so entirely preventable that Medicare, the federal health insurance program for the elderly, often will no longer pay hospitals to treat them. The hospitals have to cover the cost themselves since they could have prevented the problem in the first place. Prevention starts with screening to identify which patients are at greatest risk. The dozen or so risk factors include obesity, smoking, and surgery lasting 45 minutes or more.[23]

One option for prevention is to use blood thinning drugs to help prevent clots in the first place. A second option is to use a compression device that repeatedly squeezes patients' lower legs while they are confined to bed. A third is to get people up out of bed as soon as possible after surgery.[24]

Even though there are screening guidelines and effective methods for prevention, the incidence of these blood clots is increasing. Most people have no idea that they are at risk, and most people aren't screened or treated to prevent this problem when they are in the hospital.

One a Day

The fourth common way to die from health care is from the medicine you're given. Professionals call these situations adverse drug events. These may involve problems such as:

- the wrong drug
- the wrong dose
- a drug intended for a different patient
- a drug that interacts badly with another drug you're taking

More than 125,000 people die from adverse drug events each year,[25] as Bob almost did. These are deaths from legal drugs, not street drugs. Now, some of these deaths might not have been preventable, such as those from a previously unknown severe allergy to a drug ingredient.

But a national study mandated by the U.S. Congress concluded that 1.5 million *preventable* adverse drug events occur each year. It went on to say that "a hospital patient can expect on average to be subjected to more than one medication error each day."[26] One a day! That's a fine slogan for a vitamin; it's a disturbing one for drug errors.

Protect Yourself

It's telling that there's a whole cottage industry publishing books that advise you how to keep from being injured or killed by the health care profession. They have titles like *Protect Yourself in the Hospital*[27] and *How to Survive Your Hospital Stay*.[28] Think about that for a moment: protect yourself in the hospital?! Aren't *they* supposed to be taking care of *you*?

Even the *Journal of the American Medical Association* published an article concluding that health care is the third leading cause of death in America.[29] That study did not include all of the deaths described above. For example, it did not include deaths from blood clots. When more of the problems are captured, it becomes evident that health care is in fact the second leading cause of death, and close to tying heart disease for first place.[30]

The health care profession is trying hard to get better. Health care professionals don't come to work planning to kill people, and it's often devastating to them when they do. There's a major focus in hospitals on improving "patient safety." That slightly Orwellian turn of phrase is defined as "freedom from accidental injury due to medical care, or medical errors."[31] (Or, as Hippocrates is widely quoted as having said more than 2000 years ago, "First, do no harm.")

While there are pockets of improvement and some truly inspired initiatives,[32] there is general agreement that improvement is not happening fast enough. One article written in 2005, reporting little or no improvement from five years earlier, was titled, "To Err Is Human; To Fail to Improve Is Unconscionable."[33]

Four years after that, in 2009, a government analysis reported that patient safety was actually getting worse.[34] It's worth noting that this pattern is common in health care: a comprehensive, well-researched study identifies big problems — and five or ten years later, an update reveals that not much has changed.[35]

On a related note, many hospitals cut people and money from infection control departments in 2009.[36] Of course, many organizations have faced wide-spread cutbacks due to the economy, but this development still raises concerns. Only about half of the people who head the boards of hospitals said that quality of care was one of their top two priorities.[37]

Population of Boston

When the numbers of deaths caused by health care each year are summarized, here's what the picture looks like:

Deaths from medical errors	200,000
Deaths from hospital infections	99,000
Deaths from hospital blood clots	200,000
Deaths from adverse drug events	<u>125,000</u>
Total deaths from selected causes	624,000

Having 624,000 people die from health care gone awry is equivalent to killing off all the inhabitants of a city bigger than Boston, Massachusetts.[38] And then doing it again the following year. And the year after that. And so forth.

According to the federal government, about 2.415 million people die each year in America.[39] Doing the math (624,000/2,415,000), it's evident that nearly 26% of the deaths in this country every year happen *because* of medical care. Of course, everyone will die eventually, but these facts mean that huge numbers of people die long before they otherwise would have — in many cases, decades before.

These numbers do not include all deaths caused by medical care. They are generally considered to be understatements. They count only certain types of problems. Additionally, the studies calculating deaths from medical errors and infections focus on hospitals. They don't count medical errors or infections initiated in doctors' offices or in nursing homes.

Three Million

Consider the country's response to 9/11, with a death toll of about 3,000 people.[40] We went to war, and airports and train stations will never be the same. "Homeland Security" is a household term. Massive changes in national priorities and expectations occurred.

We've spent hundreds of billions of dollars, and about 4,300 Americans died in the first six years of combat.[41] It is widely believed that one of the reasons people voted against the incumbent party in the 2006 Congressional elections was anger over that loss of American lives.

In the last five years, the health care system in America has killed more than *three million* people. Did you even hear about that? These deaths don't happen just to the unfortunate people who don't have health insurance and can't afford appropriate care. These deaths don't take place just in poor neighborhoods. Rich or poor,[42] health care is one of the leading causes of death in the U.S.

Emergency

In addition, many more people are injured or disabled by medical care than are killed outright. As an example, one study concludes that adverse drug events outside of hospitals alone result each year in:

- 17 million trips to the emergency room
- 8 million admissions to the hospital
- 3 million admissions to long term care facilities[43]

Fifteen Million Harmed in Hospitals

A doctor wrote the following in a prestigious health policy journal:

"Three years ago my father, a longtime heart patient, had trouble breathing and complained of chest pain. He was admitted into the hospital with congestive heart failure. This is the hospital in which I have made rounds almost every day for the past three decades. . . . The CEO is my friend and patient. My father's physician is one of my young associates, well-trained and eager. I was confident that my father would receive the best medical care he could get in America today."[44]

He continued: "Yet I would not leave him alone in his hospital room. During the day, if I or my brother or mother could not be there, I had a hired sitter by his bed. . . . It is almost a miracle that any elderly patient gets out of the hospital today relatively unscathed."[45]

What is the evidence to support his conclusion?

One organization has developed a widely-used nine-level classification system, from A to I, to sort mistakes and injuries caused by health care into buckets.[46]

For example, Category F is defined as "Temporary injury from care requiring initial or prolonged hospitalization."[47] An example is someone in the hospital who falls while trying to get out of bed after a hip replacement operation, requiring additional surgery to repair damage from the fall. Falls like this are considered largely preventable. Category G is defined as "Injury from care leading to permanent patient harm." Category I results in the patient's death.[48]

Adding up Categories E through I, an analysis by the Institute for Healthcare Improvement concludes that 40% of all patients admitted to the hospital each year are then injured by the care they receive there. That's *15 million* people a year.[49]

Those numbers do not include near misses, like the drug dosing error that almost killed Bob. (That problem would fall somewhere in Categories A through D.)

Millions of people every year are newly unable, either temporarily or permanently, to lead the lives they led before they came under the care of the health care system — again, not because of the conditions that bring them there, but because of the care they are given once they arrive.

Star Trek Medicine

You may still have trouble believing that America doesn't have the best health care system in the world, because you probably know about other miracles like Bob's. How can America not be the best? The country is headed towards Star Trek medicine.

In case you missed the Star Trek craze: health care on its 24th century spaceship seemed to consist largely of running a handheld device over the body, miraculously repairing whatever internal damage had occurred.

In this century, excitement bubbles over at the potential of genomics, which includes the study of how genes impact disease. "The ultimate goal is to use this information to develop new ways to treat, cure, or even prevent the thousands of diseases that afflict humankind."[50]

On other fronts, enthusiasts say things like, "Remarkable advances in tissue regeneration and engineering hold great promise for curing diseases and prolonging life. One day, scientists and physicians may use stem cell therapies to regenerate damaged tissues and organs or to cure conditions such as Parkinson's disease, arthritis, and diabetes. They may also be used to reverse the aging process."[51]

There's only one tiny problem. It makes no difference that we've got miracles available if people die because care providers don't wash their hands. It makes no difference that we've got miracles available if people die because of medical errors. It makes no difference that we've got miracles available if people die because they're given the wrong dose of medicine.

Like Snow to Eskimos

You might be alarmed to hear that the health care profession even has specific words created to describe the harm that it can cause you:

- "Iatrogenic" means "induced in a patient by a physician's activity, manner, or therapy. Used especially of an infection or other complication of treatment."[52]
- "Nosocomial" means "of or being a secondary disorder associated with being treated in a hospital but unrelated to the patient's primary condition."[53] A "nosocomial infection" is an infection picked up in a hospital.

You may feel the way you would if you found out that your dry cleaner routinely drops your clean clothes in a mud puddle — except that people don't usually die from dirty laundry.

It's often said that Eskimos have dozens of unique words for "snow," because it's such a big part of their landscape. Think about the implications of the fact that health care providers have unique words to describe how their care can hurt you.

Good Intentions

There are millions of well-intentioned health care providers in America, and you may be someone, like me, whose life has been saved by some of them. But, like you and me, they are not infallible. They also work in a system with many, many serious problems. And those problems can kill you — or someone you care about.

Your (or a loved one's) earlier-than-necessary death or injury from medical care might happen a couple of decades down the road. But it could also happen next week or next month as a result of an unexpected close encounter with the health care system. And it doesn't have to be that way.

Social Convention

In the children's story *The Emperor's New Clothes*, the townspeople didn't believe the evidence before their own eyes. They were told that only very intelligent and capable people were able to see the emperor's fine new suit of clothes as he paraded down the street. When they looked at the naked emperor, they were embarrassed. They were certain that everyone else could see the suit.

Since they didn't want to reveal their own ignorance, they just agreed with everyone else that the suit was very fine. It took a child who relied on his own senses instead of ceding to social convention to break the spell.

Health care in America has a lot in common with *The Emperor's New Clothes*. The health care system is not what you've been led to believe it is. You can break the spell. You can understand what the major gaps are in having the health care system help you and other people you care about experience the best possible health for the longest period of time.

You have the power to make it happen.

CHAPTER TWO

Actions Speak Louder than Words

Doctors are trained to take action — write a prescription, perform surgery, and so forth — to address your health needs. However, roughly 50% of the actions they take do not help you. Many of the actions can, in fact, harm you. That outcome is not intentional, but it can create big problems for you.

Snow Boots

One February, I left Pennsylvania for a business trip to Texas. I didn't wear my heavy snow boots because I clearly wasn't going to need them in Texas. Unfortunately, that turned out to be a bad decision on my part. I slipped on ice outside my apartment, and landed directly on a knee that had already endured two operations.

I tried to ignore the pain, but a few weeks later it was too severe. Back home in Pennsylvania, I was referred to a knee doctor. He was very emphatic: "Your only choice is surgery. There is zero chance that your knee will get any better without it. You need the surgery right away. Any delay will cause further deterioration. There is nothing to discuss. There are no other options."

I asked about getting a second opinion. "You can do that," he said flatly. "Anyone else you go to will tell you exactly the same thing." My heart sank. Rehabilitation after knee surgery is, in my experience, a lengthy and painful process. The logistics of living your life are challenging too: you can't drive a car for what seems like months.

It happened that I was in the middle of being transferred to Texas. As soon as I could, I got an appointment with Dr. Michael Putney, a specialist in the small town that was my new home.

He examined me and said, "Your knee has already had so much trauma from the previous two operations. I'd hate to operate a third time. That should be the last resort." He explained to me what was causing the intense pain I was experiencing and how physical therapy could help.

I was very skeptical. "Oh, that will never work!" I said with great assurance. I was thinking, "Oh, boy, here's this small-town doctor. I'm sure the guy in the northeast is much more sophisticated and up on the latest thinking." I said, "The only option is surgery!"

Dr. Putney was very patient. "Elizabeth," he said, "what if you try physical therapy for a few weeks? If you're right and it doesn't help, then we'll go ahead with the surgery. If not, it will save you a lot of trouble. I think it's worth a shot."

"Oh, physical therapy doesn't work for me. I had a lot of it with the other two operations. They tell me to do things and I end up re-injuring the joint."

"I will send you to someone very, very good," he said. "You tell him if anything hurts and he will modify the exercise so that it doesn't."

"Okay," I sighed, reluctantly and theatrically. I concluded that the only way to get this man to do the surgery I clearly needed was to prove to him that physical therapy wouldn't work. I would keep all the PT appointments so that he couldn't claim that I hadn't tried. I would show him that he was wrong.

Three weeks passed.

He was right.

I was stunned.

I was incredulous as the pain started to decrease, and eventually I forgot what it had felt like. The doctor in Pennsylvania had been so convincing when he told me that surgery was the only option. It's been more than 15 years, and I never did have a third operation on my knee.

Unfortunately, you usually can't travel from one city to another to discover that doctors in different cities have completely different ideas about how to treat you — and that results are better in cities where treatment is less intensive (physical therapy instead of surgery, for instance).

Action for Action's Sake

Most doctors, nurses, and other health care providers are dedicated, caring professionals who genuinely want to do the right thing. They have been trained to intervene when you have a medical problem. Health care is organized to support the actions they take. Surprisingly, though, a lot of those actions do not improve your health.

Studies repeatedly report that as much as 40% of health care delivered is unnecessary or inappropriate, and accordingly not only doesn't improve health but may cause harm instead. In fact, recently some experts have concluded that the number is as high as 50%.[54]

Specialists and Hospital Beds

Your chances of having surgery if you have prostate cancer, back pain, or heart disease are six to ten times greater in some cities than in others.[55] In one case highlighting variations in practice, 63% of the children in one city had their tonsils removed, but only 7% did in a city 70 miles away.[56]

The differences in rates of surgery are not due to differences in the patients' ages, insurance coverage, and so forth. Many of the studies compare Medicare patients, the vast majority of whom are over the age of 65, and all of whom are covered by Medicare health insurance.

Some studies compare people who live as little as 30 miles apart. People with heart disease who live in the city of Elyria, Ohio are four times as likely to have angioplasty, a procedure to widen narrowed arteries to the heart, as are people in the rest of the country. They are also three times as likely to have this procedure as are similar patients in Cleveland, just 30 miles down the road.[57]

Most of the doctors in Elyria, like most doctors everywhere, are paid by the procedure. That is, the more medical procedures they perform, the more money they make. However, one health care organization in Elyria has salaried doctors in its employ. Their pay stays the same regardless of how many procedures they do. Those doctors perform angioplasty in Elyria at a rate slightly *lower* than the national average.[58]

What typically determines the rate of surgery? Is it medical necessity or the personal preference of the patients? No. What determines the rate of surgery is the number of specialists and hospital beds per person in the city.[59] The more specialists, the more surgery.[60]

And here's the kicker: when researchers compared two groups of people over the age of 65 who were equally sick at the start of the study, the people in the group that got more surgery and other treatment ended up in *worse* health than the group that got less care.[61]

What do people with a stake in delivering these treatments do when studies show that some care is unnecessary?

One federal agency which published such a report discovered the answer: "specialists quickly attacked the report, calling it flawed. One medical device maker . . . sued unsuccessfully to block its release. . . . Lawmakers [in one political party] tried to kill the agency that issued the report."[62] In other words, those with vested interests shoot the messenger.

Goldilocks and the Three Bears

But isn't the big problem with health care in America that a lot of people don't have health insurance and get too *little* care? That's certainly one problem. Too little health care isn't good for your health.[63]

Neither is too much. Health care has a lot in common with the fairy tale in which Goldilocks found one bowl of porridge too hot, one too cold, and one just right; one bed too hard, one too soft, and one just right. Like many people, you might have assumed that "more is better." With health care, it turns out, "more" is often "more likely to kill you."[64]

Imagine That

Doctors who aren't radiologists but who have x-ray equipment in their office, or own a business that does x-rays, order these tests roughly two to *eight* times as often for patients with particular conditions as do other doctors who don't have a financial interest in the testing.[65]

This situation highlights the fact that sometimes doctors who are paid by the procedure make decisions about tests and treatments in order to make money. One doctor notes, "Overconsultation and overtesting have now become facts of the medical profession. The culture is to grab patients and generate volume."

He goes on to tell of a colleague who orders at least 10 nuclear stress tests each month to help cover his costs, regardless of whether or not any of his patients actually need such a test.[66]

"Don't just stand there! Do something!"

With surprising frequency, health care providers take action even when no action is warranted. For example, according to a study published in the *Journal of the American Medical Association* and described in a *New York Times* article, almost ten million women are routinely tested for cancer "in an organ that they don't have."[67]

A Pap smear is a test for cancer of the cervix. The women in question have had their cervixes *completely removed* when they had hysterectomies for reasons other than cancer. Yet they are still having Pap smears done. No reputable organization recommends testing using Pap smear methods in this situation.[68]

Having an unnecessary Pap smear has a number of downsides. Most women do not enjoy the exam; it means taking time from work or other activities; and as a result of false positives, it can lead to needless anxiety and additional unnecessary testing and treatment.[69]

Another downside is the cost. Assume that each Pap smear, including doctor's visit and lab fees, costs $100. That's a *billion* dollars right there in wasted resources. As my mother used to say, "You can spend a dollar only once." Somebody, somewhere, is trying to figure out what health care *not* to pay for because of the money used to pay for these tests.

Wrong Diagnosis

You may assume that when doctors say, "Here's what's wrong with you," that statement is backed by certainty. They're the doctors, after all. They've studied for years and seen hundreds or thousands of patients. Surely they know what's wrong with you!

Have you seen the popular television show *House*? It features a curmudgeonly, often hostile — but brilliant — doctor who can figure out what's wrong with people when no one else can. He is permanently pain-wracked because of a disability resulting from a misdiagnosis, perhaps providing the inspiration for him to work to spare others a similar fate. The premise of the show — that doctors often don't know what's wrong with the patient — is based in fact.

Diagnostic error rates range from "1.4% in cancer biopsies to a high 20-40% misdiagnosis rate in emergency or ICU care."[70] One article reported, "autopsies uncover missed or incorrect diagnoses in up to 25 percent of hospital deaths."[71] Another reported, "Autopsy studies have shown high rates (35-40%) of missed diagnoses causing death."[72]

Yet another concluded, "Studies of autopsies have shown that doctors seriously misdiagnose fatal illnesses about 20 percent of the time. So millions of patients are being treated for the wrong disease."[73]

Another asked, "How often do autopsies turn up a major misdiagnosis in the cause of death? . . . According to three studies . . . the figure is about 40 percent [of the time]. . . . In about a third of the misdiagnoses the patients would have been expected to live if proper treatment had been administered."[74]

An article in the *Journal of the American Medical Association* in 2009 called diagnostic error the "next frontier" in patient safety.[75] ("Patient safety," as noted in Chapter One, means not damaging patients as they proceed through the health care system.)

The *American Journal of Medicine* published an entire supplement titled "Diagnostic Error: Is Overconfidence the Problem?" It suggests that diagnostic errors occur 10-15% of the time.[76]

Regardless of which studies and which numbers you choose to focus on, it's clear that diagnostic error is a huge problem. Said another way, doctors often embark on treatments without knowing what is wrong, so of course the treatments in those cases are unlikely to help.

Tools to help improve diagnoses are available, but they aren't often used. One of these is a computer program named Isabel,[77] which might be considered an electronic version of Dr. House, minus the limp and the attitude.

Isabel was created as a result of one father's experience in which his three-year-old daughter Isabel nearly died as a result of misdiagnosis. One study showed that using Isabel resulted in important changes in diagnosis 14% of the time.[78]

Explaining the problem of misdiagnosis, one article points out, "Under the current medical system, doctors, nurses, lab technicians and hospital executives are not actually paid to come up with the right diagnosis. They are paid to perform tests and to do surgery and to dispense drugs."[79]

Ready, Fire, Aim

Most health treatments — even operations that cost $50,000 — help only about half the people who get them. It is logical to conclude that the health care system prizes treating people, independent of whether the treatment actually improves their health. The next chapter helps explain why.

CHAPTER THREE

"Enough about me. Let's talk about you.
What do *you* think of me?"

Surprisingly, health care isn't about helping you enjoy the best health possible. Health care is not about you. It's about doctors.[80] There are logical reasons why the health care system has this perspective, but it creates challenges for you.

It's Not about You

Most of the problems with health care in America today stem from one simple and outrageous fact: *health care is not about you.*

- It does not have as a goal optimizing your chances for a long and healthy life.
- It does not typically recognize you as even an equal partner in your own health care. Even less often does it consider the possibility that you might want to be the one making decisions.

You already know that your life expectancy is shorter than that of people in other developed nations. You already know that you're at risk for medical errors, hospital-acquired infections, blood clots, and adverse drug events. But what happens long before your situation gets that serious? A great deal is known about what care is important to help people stay healthy or to save their lives in the long run.

Too Little

The previous chapter discussed the fact that doctors over use care that they get paid well to execute: performing more surgery than is warranted, ordering lots of diagnostic tests when they own the testing service, and so forth.

But they don't always do too much. They often do too little. How can that be? The things they do too little of tend to be low tech, boring, elementary things. Some of these involve coaching the patient rather than executing something interesting themselves. Here are examples of under used care:

- Only 64% of the elderly who went to the doctor were offered a vaccine which could help prevent 10,000 deaths from pneumonia each year.
- Only 61% of people with heart attacks are prescribed aspirin, even though it reduces by 15% - 40% the risk of deaths, more heart attacks, and strokes.
- Only 24% of people with diabetes had the most useful kind of test of their blood sugar levels — a test considered essential to help manage the disease to avoid blindness, kidney failure, and amputations.
- Only 18% of smokers with severe breathing problems were counseled that they would be better off not smoking.[81]

Doctors deliver appropriate care like these basics, recommended in widely accepted guidelines, only 55% of the time.[82]

The big, national, well-respected study which drew that conclusion went on to say, "Virtually everyone in this country is at risk for poor care. . . . Findings shatter the widely held perception that health care quality is not a problem in the United States. . . . Deficiencies in care . . . pose serious threats to the health of the American public. . . . There is a tremendous gap between what we know works and what patients are actually getting."[83]

Or as another report said, "Preventive measures, like a daily dose of aspirin, colon cancer screening and smoking-cessation therapy, are all effective ways to save lives and healthcare dollars, but fewer than half of Americans who need these services are getting them."[84]

Why does this omission occur? Because *health care isn't designed to help people achieve good health.* It's designed to deliver tests and treatments. In fact, an international study involving nineteen countries showed that the U.S. ranked dead last in preventing preventable deaths.[85] These generally are deaths from chronic conditions — deaths that happen precisely because preventive actions like those mentioned above aren't taken.

Thermometers

One pilot project discovered that teaching low-income parents simple things like how to use a thermometer to check their children's fevers cut emergency room visits by nearly 50%.[86] "Medicaid could save billions of dollars annually if low-income parents are trained how to better handle minor childhood ailments such as sore throats, fevers and runny noses."[87]

"These training sessions, which involve just a few hours' worth of sessions spread over the course of a couple weeks, give parents enough confidence to handle situations instead of rushing to outside help."[88]

People make 119 million trips to emergency rooms each year.[89] The nation's emergency rooms are dangerously overcrowded. It's a crisis. And it's possible to cut visits by some groups in half just by helping them understand how to do simple things themselves so they can be more self-reliant? Yes.

So why doesn't the health care system help people help themselves? *It doesn't see patients or their family members as part of the equation.* Instead of coaching people so that they don't use emergency rooms when they don't need to, health care professionals create many complicated initiatives to address overcrowding in the ER.

Yesterday's Problems

Probably, every doctor and nurse you know has good intentions. So why does health care focus so much on delivering treatments rather than on getting good results?

Excellent question.

Health care is organized to solve the health problems of a prior era, one in which it didn't need to be about you in order to get good results. Now it does, but the health care system hasn't caught on to this fact yet. Consider three eras in health care in the last hundred years.

In the first era, a hundred years ago, people usually died of infectious diseases. Big improvements in health came from cleaning up the water supply and improving sewage treatment.

The people who drove those actions were trained professionals working in public health agencies.[90] (Public health agencies address issues that affect entire communities. Examples of their responsibilities are ensuring a safe water supply and monitoring environmental hazards.[91])

Individuals didn't even have to know about these activities, to benefit. And life expectancy increased *21 years* (from 47 years for people born at the turn of the century to 68 years for people born in 1950[92]) — a huge leap.

In the second era, in the middle of the last century, people still died of infectious diseases and other sudden-onset problems. They were just much older when they succumbed, compared to people in the previous era. Improvements in health came from *acute interventions* for *acute conditions.*

Acute conditions are those that arise suddenly. Infections are typical examples. Broken bones and allergic reactions to bee stings are other examples. Acute conditions need to be treated promptly. Penicillin, vaccinations,[93] and surgery can all be considered *acute interventions* — treatments given once or over a short period of time.

In this second era, doctors like those in Norman Rockwell paintings took the actions needed to improve health. Again, these were trained professionals. They had studied medicine for years. Taking these actions was their job, eight or ten or twelve hours a day.

Individuals in this era did have to do something: they had to show up. But that's about all. They might not have known what their diagnosis was. They might not have known much about what their treatment was.

They put their lives in the hands of Marcus Welby, M.D. — the kindly general practitioner who solved every problem and healed every ill. And life expectancy continued to rise — not as much as in the previous 50 years, but it still went up 9 years[94] between 1950 and the year 2000.

Meet the CEO

The third era is today. With the great and continuing successes of the prior two eras, you could say that we now have the "luxury" of dying of chronic diseases. A chronic disease is something that usually develops slowly and can last a long time, like diabetes or heart disease. Chronic diseases typically aren't cured. Instead, the idea is either to prevent them or to manage them to reduce their harm.

Today, 70% of all deaths in this country are due to chronic conditions, not acute conditions like infectious diseases.[95] What counts most in preventing or managing chronic conditions are the actions people take every day in five areas: diet, exercise, alcohol, tobacco, and, interestingly enough, stress management.[96]

People go to the doctor on average 4 times a year.[97] What drives their health is largely what they do the other 361 days a year, in a dozen decisions every day.

It's whether they go for a bicycle ride or sit in front of a computer playing video games. It's whether they order the small ice cream cone or the triple-decker. It's whether they fume endlessly about their boss or find a constructive way to manage their stress.

Considering the common chronic diseases, it becomes clear that *doctors cannot make good health happen.* They can't snatch the potato chips off your lunch tray. They can't drag you up off the couch after dinner so that you go for a walk instead of watching old *Law & Order* reruns. They're not there.

The people who have to take the actions necessary to improve health in this era are rank amateurs: 300 million people — the entire population of the U.S. Most of them are not trained health care professionals. Working to improve health isn't their day job. Yet to get good outcomes in this era, they need to be CEOs of their own health and health care.

This arrangement is not working. The *New England Journal of Medicine* published an article which forecasted that life expectancy in the U.S. may drop by up to *five years*.[98] The projected drop is due largely to the increase in obesity and the related rise in diabetes.

The idea that life expectancy in the U.S. can drop is an affront to our sense of how things are supposed to work. Life is supposed to get better with each succeeding generation, not worse.

The Center of Attention

The health care system still acts as if it is operating in the era of the Norman Rockwell doctor. In that era, supporting doctors in delivering acute interventions was equivalent to improving health. Dying of pneumonia? The doctor gave a shot of penicillin. Polio a threat? The doctor administered the vaccine.

That arrangement worked quite well. Huge advances have been made — and continue to be made — in acute care. However, a focus on doctors delivering acute interventions has also meant that:

- Medical errors, hospital-acquired infections, blood clots, and adverse drug events are tolerated as part of the landscape.
- Interventions that don't improve health, such as excessive surgery and tests, are rampant.
- Omissions of simple, basic care that can improve your health or save your life are commonplace.

Today, the three problems above — potentially fatal flaws in health care delivery, over use of high-tech treatments, and under use of low-tech screening, coaching, and treatment — are often accepted as by-products of having doctors deliver acute interventions.

To improve health in this era, the focus of health care needs to change. The health care system needs to make you the center of attention. It needs to support you in your role as CEO of your own health and health care. But it hasn't made that shift yet. Here is an example.

Tuberculosis and Diabetes

Type II diabetes, the most common kind of diabetes, is a chronic disease whose existence and course are largely determined by how attentive people are to managing their diet, exercising, monitoring their own blood sugar levels, and so forth.

It's a disease that isn't resolved by doctors' writing a prescription or giving a shot. It requires persistent attention, every day, from the person who has diabetes. It's a huge challenge to manage well. People with diabetes need lots of coaching and guidance to pull it off.

In the New York City public health system, as of 2006, three people and less than a million dollars a year were allocated to try to deal with diabetes, which affects about a million people in the city. That's about a dollar per person with this potentially deadly disease.[99]

At the same time, tuberculosis, with 1,000 patients a year, got 400 staffers and $27 million dollars. That's $27,000 dollars per person. That's 27,000 times as much for a traditional infectious disease as for a chronic disease.[100]

Tuberculosis is a serious disease and preventing the spread of dangerous infectious diseases is important. However, there are certainly many more people dying today in New York as a result of complications of diabetes than from tuberculosis.

The staggering discrepancy in resources makes sense if you look at it as an example of a system still organized around yesterday's problems. The health care system is pretty good at controlling the traditional infectious diseases in this country. It's pretty good at monitoring water quality and — with enough lead time — at providing vaccines and penicillin and so forth.

What it's *not* good at is organizing health care around *you,* making health care work and getting good outcomes when the person who has to take action every day isn't the public health service and isn't the doctor, but instead is *you.*

Foot Work

More than 100,000 people in the U.S. have a foot or leg amputated each year for reasons other than accidents. Most of these are people with diabetes.[101] Researchers estimate that almost 85% of those amputations could be avoided.

"'Any amputation, especially for conditions like diabetes, is a human tragedy and a gross failure of public health efforts,' said Dr. Robert Beaglehole, W.H.O.'s director of chronic diseases and health promotion. 'We are failing desperately to prevent the most preventable conditions.'"[102] Often, individuals are not even on the radar screen at all until they deteriorate to the point that an infection becomes life-threatening, and then doctors cut off their legs.

Why aren't these amputations prevented?

An amputation is an intervention a *surgeon* can execute. If you have diabetes, getting you a special thermometer for checking the temperature of your feet every day and training you to do it[103]— a way to tell if an infection is brewing in time to prevent it from causing serious harm — puts *you* in the driver's seat with an intervention you can execute.

That arrangement is not something the health care system supports very well. Granted, it's not easy to do. Many individuals don't realize that they have a central role to play, and it takes a lot of work to help them do it right. But that just means that the health care system needs to try harder.

Even if it's gotten to the point where surgery is required, there are usually choices about whether to amputate or not. An alternative is surgery that improves the flow of blood to the leg or foot, which can make it possible for the infected body part to heal. Here's what one doctor had to say about that choice: "Doctors have to decide whether to spend three or four hours doing a complicated salvage procedure, or 35 minutes for a short, quick amputation."[104]

That doesn't sound like a focus on getting the best outcome for the individual. It sounds like a focus on the surgeon, and maximizing the number of surgeries he can perform in a day. What happens next isn't individual-centric either: about 70% of people with diabetes who have a foot or leg amputated die within five years.[105]

On Stage

One reason that health care doesn't work as well as it might is that there's a glaring mismatch between the nature of the problem today — chronic disease — and the nature of the solutions being applied — acute treatments.

It probably makes sense to treat many acute conditions — for example, injuries from automobile accidents — with acute solutions. But for most chronic diseases, there's plenty of time up front to apply what might be called chronic preventions. And failing that, to apply chronic management. But that's not what usually happens.

The nature of the problem has shifted, so that *you* need to be the principal actor, 365 days a year, and the doctor needs to be the supporting actor, showing up onstage and in the spotlight much less frequently than you do. This role reversal is hard for the medical profession to adapt to. In fact, even when doctors think that they are being empathetic and supportive of patients, it turns out that they're often simply turning the spotlight on themselves.

A recent study "showed that many doctors waste patients' time and lose their focus in office visits by interjecting irrelevant information about themselves."[106] It went on to say, "There was no evidence that any of the doctors' disclosures about themselves helped patients or established rapport." The doctors doing the study commented, "We were quite shocked. . . . Most of the time self-disclosure had more to do with us than with the patients."[107]

Sound Bites

Prevention is supported very well by the health care system when professionals deliver it. Two examples are injecting vaccines and cleaning your teeth. However, when the main actor needs to be you, it's a different story. The advice you do get about actions *you* take — eating, for instance — is often unintentionally designed and delivered in a way that makes it wildly unlikely that you can actually follow it.

Consider the experience of a food critic and journalist in excellent health who decided to eat for just four days according to the guidelines published by the U.S. Department of Agriculture. (That framework is commonly referred to as the food pyramid.) In his entertaining article titled, "Eating My Spinach: Four Days on the Uncle Sam Diet,"[108] William Grimes chronicles his failed attempt to figure out how to construct plausible meals consistent with the guidelines. After two days, he notes, "The guidelines were beginning to feel like wartime rationing."

His wife neatly captures their conclusion: "No one is ever going to eat like this."[109] That is, the government has told 300 million people to eat in a way that was impossible for someone who had the necessary cooking skills, money, time, and motivation. Where does that leave the rest of us?

There are many things for you to do to prevent most chronic conditions — eat right, be physically active, not use tobacco, and so forth. And the "help" you get for most of these may consist largely of exhortations: "Lose weight!" "Exercise more!" Health care by exhortation has been a notorious failure.[110] For example, it is commonly thought that only about 5% - 10% of people who lose weight succeed in keeping it off.[111]

The fact that there's a 90-95% failure rate is a hint that health care isn't actually focused on helping you get good results. By way of analogy, if a few students fail a class, one tends to think that they all have deficiencies of some kind. But if 90-95% of the students fail, one has to suspect that the *teacher* is falling short.

Many people argue that the issues with weight management are beyond the abilities of individuals and their doctors to address. They note that obesity is linked to changes in our environment: "Parents are working longer, and takeout meals have become a default dinner. Gym classes have been cut. The real price of soda has fallen 33 percent over the last three decades. The real price of fruit and vegetables has risen more than 40 percent. The solutions to these problems are beyond the control of any individual."[112]

What is needed, many observers conclude, is a larger public health effort focused on obesity and other contributors to chronic diseases. If that's what is needed most to improve health, why isn't that where the time, money, and effort is going? One possible answer is that getting good health outcomes for you isn't the main focus. Instead, delivering acute interventions is the focus.

Patience, Patients

Even the words used to label you may suggest that you and your best interests aren't the priority. Consider the term "patient." Here are its dictionary definitions:

- "bearing or enduring pain, difficulty, provocation or annoyance with calmness"
- "one who receives medical attention, care, or treatment"[113]

It might be interesting to learn why the same word has both of these meanings. However, that's a topic for another day. Consider instead just the second definition.

Who wants to be a *patient*? Most people just want to be *people*, leading their lives. Being a patient implies being sick, which most people find to be a huge and unwelcome disruption to their regular lives. If they are sick, they just want the illness to be over with so they can get back to normal. If they have a chronic condition, then dealing with it has to be part of their *normal* lives.

They want to focus on their families, their jobs, their friends, and so forth. They don't want their lives to be about doctors and medical treatments. Calling them patients emphasizes the illness. It puts them in a box in which being sick defines them. Who wants that?

Doctors, apparently. David Shore of Harvard tells about the reaction of some high-powered doctors who were required to attend two days of "customer service" training, in an attempt to get them to be more responsive to the needs of the people they were treating. The doctors were outraged by the very idea, and returned to the second day of the mandatory workshop sporting buttons that read, "Prostitutes have customers. Doctors have patients."[114]

The Health Care Consumer

Another common term is "consumers." According to the dictionary, a consumer is "one that consumes."[115] That's not the best idea for health care. (Buy, buy, buy!) As discussed in Chapter Two, getting more health care can sometimes be fatal.

There's been a remarkable and unnoticed coup driven by marketers in the past few decades. Marketers are the people who dream up ways to get you to buy toothpaste, cereal, computer services, automobiles, airplane tickets, and thousands of other products and services. Here's the coup: 300 million people, with all of their intellectual, social, emotional, physical, and spiritual dimensions, have ceased being "people" and are routinely referred to in the media as "consumers."

Calling you "patient" puts doctors in charge. Calling you "consumer" puts marketers in charge. It would be reasonable to ask whether either of these suggests a health care system with a focus on your best interests. Although it's a challenge to break away from the common lingo, this book will at times refer to people seeking help from the health care system simply as "people" or "individuals."

CHAPTER FOUR

The Patient as Footnote

Professionals designing how health care will work often neglect to consider the impact of their designs on your well-being. Often, simple and inexpensive changes that could make a huge difference for you are not even considered.

Bright Lights

Where would you find an environment with characteristics like these?

- Individuals' personal belongings, such as clothing, are removed.
- People have little information about, or control over, what is happening.
- They are in pain, and are physically restrained.
- Bright lights shine on them 24/7, but there are no windows.
- Frequent, loud, intermittent noises occur around the clock.
- As a result of the lights and noise, they are seriously disoriented. They are unable to tell if it is night or day, and they are extremely sleep deprived.

Where would you find that environment? The same two accurate answers have surfaced in every audience asked this question: first, a prison camp for terrorist suspects; second, a hospital ICU (Intensive Care Unit).[116] Think about that for a moment.

Additionally, people in an ICU have two big strikes against them that prisoners don't. First, they are very, very sick when they arrive. Second, they almost certainly are drugged, which terrorist suspects typically are not.[117]

What happens to people in an ICU as a result of being subjected to an environment with a lot of characteristics in common with those created in prison camps to break people? A third of them develop ICU Psychosis, in as little as 24 hours.[118] In lay terms, they are driven insane. They start hallucinating. They experience a complete psychotic break from reality.

In medical terms, this experience is described as "a form of delirium, or acute brain failure."[119] It's described as "psychotic episode(s) occurring within 24 hours after entering the ICU in patients with no previous history of psychosis."[120]

Doctors typically respond to concerned family members shocked by a relative's sudden irrationality by saying, "Oh, don't worry, that's completely normal. It happens to everybody in the ICU. Once they're out of the hospital, they'll be fine."[121]

That assurance doesn't square with the facts. In the six months following an ICU stay, people who developed ICU Psychosis die at three times the rate of people who were equally sick who did not develop ICU Psychosis.[122]

Even if they survive, people who developed ICU Psychosis often experience serious long-term consequences such as post-traumatic stress disorder[123] or permanent cognitive decline. The outcome may be that they never go home again — not as a result of the condition that put them in the ICU, but as a result of the ICU Psychosis induced once they got there.[124]

ICU Psychosis is considered easy to prevent,[125] and the actions required do not interfere with medical treatment. One simple example is that dimming the lights at night goes a long way toward keeping people oriented. But such actions are rarely taken. Why is that?

Doctors, nurses, and hospital administrators do not wake up in the morning and say, "I'm going to find ways to damage more people today." They don't think that way any more than you do. It is not intentional that conditions in a typical ICU are massively destructive. Those conditions exist simply because the health care system often doesn't consider the cumulative or long-term impact of its actions on you.

It doesn't consider these things because it still thinks the way it did when improving your health meant delivering an acute intervention for an acute condition. For example, the benefits of giving you a shot of penicillin to cure your pneumonia clearly outweighed any potential downsides: if you didn't get the shot, you'd die.

Today, the health care system is delivering a lot of *acute* interventions for *chronic* conditions. The interventions are more complicated, more invasive, and are a bigger assault on your body than were many of the interventions fifty years ago for acute conditions.

The health care system hasn't recognized this gradual shift. Its thinking about the impact of its interventions on you is fifty years out of date. It acts as if the only impacts are the ones it intends, and doesn't really look beyond those to discover that there are impacts it didn't intend or impacts that surface over time.

The example of ICU Psychosis is used as shorthand in a number of places in the rest of this book. It is used to represent the thousands of ways in which health care fails to be individual-centric.

"I can't believe you'd insult me like this!"

The lack of attention to bad consequences that can result from treatments isn't limited to hospitals. *Prevention* magazine chronicles the story of a woman who, like millions of the elderly, was prescribed several drugs.[126] After she started taking them, she developed new symptoms, so more drugs were prescribed. Then she developed more symptoms, so yet more drugs were added, and so forth, until she was taking 13 drugs.

She reached the point where she felt so awful that she wanted to die. She asked a pharmacist to analyze her drug regimen. He identified a number of drug interactions and known side effects that were probably causing most of her problems.

And here's the interesting part:

She went to her doctor, and gave him the pharmacist's carefully researched report. Her doctor said, "I can't believe you'd insult me like this!" and threw the report across the room at her. He ended the visit, and later sent her a registered letter telling her to find another doctor.

Notice that the central issue to the doctor was what he perceived as a challenge to his authority, something so unacceptable that he fired the patient.

The next *eight* doctors that she went to, in an attempt to get her drug regimen changed, refused to consider the idea that the drugs might be causing her symptoms. Some of them got very angry at the suggestion.

That reaction makes sense if you realize that doctors subconsciously believe that interventions — treatments — are the *purpose* of health care. That's engrained in them. It's so much a part of them, it's like breathing. Suggesting that the drugs were *causing* her problems bordered on heresy.

The *tenth* doctor agreed to work with her, and reduced her drug regimen from 13 drugs to 3 drugs. "Within a week, [the woman] felt substantially better, and within a month she was back to her old self. These days, she takes three prescription drugs, a daily aspirin, and a few vitamins and minerals — and feels 15 years younger."[127]

Here's a similar story: "Recently, my mother, 94, lay slowly dying. She was skeletal, feeble, disoriented, delusional and agitated, and she slept fitfully. She took water by medicine dropper and refused all food. . . . Three days later, although still occasionally confused, she sat at the kitchen table requesting pancakes for breakfast and making sharp-witted remarks. Two weeks later, her mental condition and energy level were essentially normal for the first time in years."

What turned her life around? Her son's insistence that she stop being given so many drugs.[128]

These stories are very, very common. Usually, though, they do not have a good outcome. Usually they end very badly, particularly with the elderly.

According to one study, "polypharmacy," as the prescribing of multiple drugs is called, is responsible for up to 28% of hospital admissions.[129] Thirty-seven million people are admitted to the hospital each year.[130] These numbers mean that millions and millions of people land in the hospital every year as a result of being prescribed too many conflicting drugs.

A study done seven years earlier, quoted in Chapter One, put the number of hospital admissions each year from all adverse drug events at 8 million, including those related to a bad reaction to just one drug.

For this discussion, it doesn't matter what the precise number of adverse drug events is, or exactly how it breaks down between problems caused by one drug and problems caused by combinations of drugs. No matter how you analyze the data, the result is a big number.

Why are so many people made so sick that they have to go to the hospital due to the combination of drugs they are given? It is reasonable to conclude that it happens because the focus of the health care system is on delivering interventions, not necessarily on getting good outcomes for people.

Grades and Curves

In ways large and small, people routinely run up against the fact that what they need from health care in order to feel better often isn't even on the radar screen. Here's a story of the aftermath of a bicycle accident:

It was the first nice Saturday in weeks, and I had set off early in the morning on my bicycle. Because I liked the freedom to pursue unfamiliar routes, my bike bag held maps of seven counties and four bottles of water. I committed only to getting home in time for dinner.

After ten or fifteen miles, I didn't recognize the road, and got out a map to plot my course. Unfortunately, the map wasn't topographical, and I soon found myself in the ignominious position of having to get off and push the bike up an awfully steep and apparently endless hill. When I finally reached the top, I saw signs with pictures of trucks slanting downwards on triangles, and the notation "15% grade."

I was briefly curious, but generally oblivious. The sun was shining, birds were singing, and a gentle breeze was blowing. And I certainly wasn't going to walk *down* a hill when I had just walked *up* the other side. There had to be some reward for all that effort!

The road had lots of curves. It was impossible to see where it went. I assumed that it would level out shortly. I thought it had to — there was a big highway that I realized must be at the bottom of the hill, half a mile away and out of sight. I knew that it had no overpass or underpass; it had only a stop light between me and tractor-trailers barreling along at 70 mph.

I folded up the map and got on the bike. Very soon, I was startled to realize that I was going faster than I'd ever ridden. Much, much faster. The brakes were clearly a laughable little toy with not a chance of stopping me now. And those semis were not far away.

I very gently squeezed the brakes. I came to a sharp curve and hit a patch of gravel, and the bike wobbled. Then I hit the ground. I bounced and rolled, bounced and rolled, and bounced and rolled again. When I came to a stop, I was on my back, looking up at the sky, one foot on the curb.

I knew, since I could feel the curb, that I probably wasn't in danger of being run over. I knew I'd broken my wrist. I suspected there was other damage as well. I hurt in many places. I wondered if I could ride home ten miles with a broken wrist. Then I thought, "Maybe I'll just lie here for a moment before I figure out what to do next."

The first person who leapt out of her car and came racing over was an ER nurse. The second was an ex-cop. The third was an off-duty paramedic. I felt like I was in a sitcom: an ER nurse, an ex-cop, and a paramedic, within 60 seconds?! I thought, "Okay, maybe I'll let *them* figure out what to do next."

Later, the policeman who responded to the 911 call looked at the computer on my bicycle and told me that I'd been going 44 mph when I crashed.

Damages

"If your wife hadn't been wearing a bicycle helmet, you wouldn't be standing here talking to her. You'd be making funeral arrangements," the emergency room nurse said to my husband. We were in a curtained cubicle where I lay strapped to a backboard with a big foam collar around my neck, just like on the television show *ER*.

After six hours in the emergency room, here was the tally:

- Broken right wrist.
- Left arm flayed raw from elbow to wrist; also some puncture wounds from pieces of gravel half an inch in diameter, embedded so far that no one realized they were there for the first five hours.
- Massive hematoma on my left hip. A hematoma is caused by a blood vessel breaking and bleeding (quite a lot, in this case) into the surrounding tissue. It looked as if I'd attached half a honeydew melon to my side.
- Extensive abrasions — "road rash" — on my right thigh and both knees.

Gauze Pads

Given all of these injuries, what caused me the most pain and greatest subsequent trauma? The gauze pads they prescribed in the emergency room.

From my left arm, layers of skin had disappeared into the asphalt. When I moved my arm, it felt as if it were the inside of an hourglass filled with little shards of glass and turned upside down. Something very painful was pouring through my arm every time I moved it.

They explained to my husband and me that he would have to change the many gauze pads twice a day to avoid infection. The first time we tried this, we were incredulous. Every bit of healing tissue stuck to the gauze and was ripped off my arm, accompanied by excruciating pain.

The next day, my husband said as he tried to change the bandage, "We have to stop. You've gone chalk white. You're going to pass out." We called the doctor and asked for an appointment, explaining that:

- My arm hurt more.
- It felt more swollen and hot.
- We couldn't get the gauze off, and surely my arm would never heal if we kept ripping off all the new tissue every time we changed the bandage.

The doctor's office refused to give me an appointment. "We don't change dressings," they said dismissively. We begged and pleaded and after several phone calls, a clearly irritated staff member grudgingly agreed that I could come in.

The doctor and nurse again chastised me for asking them to do something that they felt my husband should have done for me. Then they pulled the gauze off, again ripping away all the new tissue. The pain was again excruciating. A senior physician was brought in to check the work of the junior staffer before they re-bandaged my arm.

He asked a few questions. Then he took a closer look, and said, "This arm is infected." He prescribed antibiotics and had turned to leave when I again blurted out that ripping the healing tissue off twice a day couldn't be good. He looked at me quizzically and said, "If the gauze is sticking, use Teflon-coated gauze pads. They won't stick."

"WHAT?!" my husband and I said simultaneously. "Where do you get them? What are they called?" He told us, we bought some, and the horrible, hour-long, twice-daily trauma was history. Just like that.

The health care system had opportunities to give us this information earlier: in the emergency room when they gave us instructions for what to do at home, and when we called the doctor's office and told the triage nurse that the gauze was ripping the skin off.

For lack of this information — a few seconds, a few words — and lack of the correct product, I had:

- suffered through many hours of excruciating pain
- gotten an infection, perhaps aided by all the time-consuming handling (it had taken up to an hour to change the bandage each time, partly because we had been instructed to soak the arm to try to get the bandage to loosen) and re-opening of the wound by repeatedly ripping off all the new skin
- had to have several additional office visits
- needed to take very powerful antibiotics
- had to take potent painkillers for longer than I would otherwise have had to
- ended up with what was probably more severe permanent scarring

Why hadn't they said anything? It's standard in health care to think about the actions the *doctor* takes. Changing bandages was something *we* were to do. Consequently, it was not given much thought.

Remote Control

Many hospital rooms are now being designed for one person instead of for two people.[131] It was recently discovered that patients who have peace and quiet — some control over visitors, the television, and the lights — heal much faster and have fewer complications.[132]

This fact is not a surprise to anyone who has stayed in a hospital. People often have horror stories about being kept up all night by the moaning of the person in the next bed, or being unable to rest during the day because the other person's television was always on.

Why is it only now that hospitals are starting to act on this knowledge? It is because historically their focus was on what doctors and nurses needed in order to deliver treatments. Little thought was given to what you needed in order to heal.

You've Got Mail. . . . Not!

Individuals use e-mail regularly for business and personal communication. Studies repeatedly show that most people would like to be able to communicate with their doctors by e-mail, especially for simple things like getting prescription renewals and following up on minor problems.[133]

Yet one study reported that only 16.6% of doctors had *ever* used e-mail to communicate with patients, and only 2.9% reported doing so frequently. They use e-mail with family and with other doctors; just not with patients.[134] A newer study reports that 31% of doctors use e-mail with patients; it's not clear if they do so regularly, or simply that they have done it occasionally.[135]

Doctors are doing what they want instead of what their customers (that's you) want. For example, one study notes that "68% of PCPs [primary care providers] preferred telephone communication for routine follow-up of minor medical problems compared with 26% of patients." Doctors preferred written communication (snail mail) for test results 44% of the time; patients only 7%.[136]

The issue isn't security — the technical issues are addressable. One of the objections doctors have to using e-mail? It is that "the art of medicine might be marginalized."[137]

That doesn't sound like a health care system that's about you.

CHAPTER FIVE

The Mushroom Treatment

You are often kept in the dark about how likely it is that a proposed treatment will actually help you, and about what kinds of problems it might cause you. Doctors rarely provide this basic information, and instead often expect that you will simply follow their instructions. This approach endangers your health and well-being.

Treatment

One year, I had a DEXAscan, a test to see if my bones were thinning. It turns out that the prescription for the test was based on an error in the doctor's office. According to her records, I had shrunk two inches between visits. My husband started laughing when I told him about this latest medical evaluation. "Not unless I've also shrunk two inches," he said. "You still fit under my chin exactly as you always have."

Subsequent measurements proved him correct. In the meantime, I had the test. I couldn't see what harm a simple diagnostic test could have, so I didn't push back. The doctor called me after she got the test results and prescribed a drug. Call the prescription Drug A. It was heavily marketed by the drug company that sells it.

A month later, I returned to the doctor with severe pain in my buttocks. The doctor added prescriptions for Drugs B and C. A month after that, the pain was so severe that I was entirely unable to ride my bicycle or even swim. I felt disabled. Dealing with a typical day in the office was very difficult. Business travel was agonizing. The doctor sent me for hip x-rays to see if I had somehow broken my hip. I had not.

The doctor doubled the dose of Drug C. Four months later, with the pain still severe, she added two more drugs, D and E, to the treatment regimen. I had entirely stopped exercising due to the pain. I had gained weight. In the following two months, I had ten visits to a chiropractor for back pain.

The next month, I had such severe gastrointestinal pain that I was unable to eat anything at all for about a week. Around the same time, I reviewed my care with a highly skilled doctor, an internist I was lucky enough to have had access to at work.

He was startled that I had been prescribed *any* drug based on the DEXAscan: my test results did not fall into the range for which the drug was considered appropriate. He recommended stopping all five drugs. I did so. Within a few weeks, all of the excruciating pain and disruptive disability were history.

In the years following, reports surfaced about side effects of the five drugs the doctor had prescribed for me, explaining all of the nearly year-long distress I had experienced. One of the drugs, in fact, was subsequently taken off the market.

A follow up DEXAscan a year after that showed that my bones had in fact strengthened. The drug had worked. But that gain essentially cost me a year of my life. If I had understood at any point that it was the cause of my suffering — in conjunction with the four drugs added to deal with the harm it was causing me — I would never have taken it.

Two Questions

When the doctor prescribes a treatment for you, two questions you might have regarding its impact on your health are:

- Does it solve my problem?
- Does it create other problems?

Those two questions suggest four possible outcomes, as shown in Figure 1. For the sake of illustration, assume that the treatment in question is a drug to treat a chronic condition.

Best Box

The box in the upper right is a great place to be: the drug solves your original problem and doesn't create any others. That is an excellent result.

However, across the health care industry, data suggest that on average, only about 50% of the people benefit from any particular treatment. That fact means that the other 50% fall in one of the two boxes in the bottom half of the chart.

Three Other Boxes

In the bottom right-hand box the drug doesn't help, but it doesn't cause any serious side effects either. That doesn't sound so bad. But if individuals are being treated because their condition requires it, and the drug isn't working for them, presumably they are likely to get sicker. Additionally, a great deal of money is being spent without yielding any benefit. That money then can't be spent on more useful things.

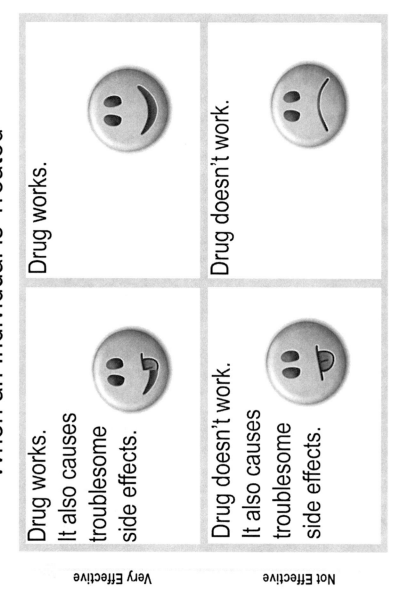

When an Individual is Treated

Drug works.

Drug works.
It also causes
troublesome
side effects.

Drug doesn't work.

Drug doesn't work.
It also causes
troublesome
side effects.

Very Effective

Not Effective

Side Effects

No Side Effects

Figure 1

More than 4 *billion* prescriptions are written every year in the U.S. — nearly 15 for every man, woman, and child in the country.[138] They cost $270 billion dollars.[139] If 50% of the time the drugs don't work for people, then roughly $135 billion dollars are being wasted. The bottom right-hand box is not a great place to be.

In the bottom left-hand box, the situation is even worse. Here, the drug not only doesn't solve the original problem, it also creates new ones. For example, many drugs are known to cause significant weight gain in many of the people who take them. That alone can cause serious health problems.

In the upper left-hand box, life gets complicated. Here the drug solves the original problem — and creates other problems. That was the case for me in the example above. Here, the best option is for doctors to work closely with people for whom they've prescribed the drugs. They can adjust the dosing and make other changes in an attempt to reduce side effects while still producing most of the benefits of treatment. That's often very tough to pull off.

Focus on One Box

Every person taking any drug will land in one of these four boxes. In only one of those boxes should individuals almost certainly be encouraged to continue taking the medicine. The half of the people who fall into the bottom two boxes shouldn't be taking the drug at all, and many of the people in the upper left box shouldn't either.

However, it is very common in health care for professionals to talk and act as if there is only one box: the one in the upper right, where only good things happen. Here's what one insurance company wrote to its enrollees: "Taking medicine is an important part of staying healthy. It's very important to take your medicine exactly as ordered."[140]

On a similar note, a doctor writing in a prestigious medical journal opined, "Our success or failure in combating osteoporosis increasingly depends not so much on the drugs available to us but rather on our ability to engage our patients and ensure that they take the medicines we prescribe."[141]

Researchers at the Mayo Clinic discovered that after people went home from the hospital with new drug prescriptions, "only 11% reported that they had been told of potential adverse effects."[142] Other research similarly concluded that "providers often neglected to tell patients about the potential disadvantages of treatments or tests that they recommended."[143]

Thus, when health care professionals talk about you and prescription drugs, they tend to talk about coming up with the right carrots and sticks to drive you to take the drugs that doctors have prescribed for you. They call this idea "compliance" or "adherence."

Given that there are *four* boxes on the chart, it becomes obvious that your health is more likely to improve not as a result of your simply following doctors' orders, but instead by your taking a more active role: as CEO of your own health and health care, figuring out which box you fall into.

CEO's Questions

CEOs don't know everything. They rely heavily on experts, all of whom know more about their field of expertise than the CEO does. What the CEO does know is what questions to ask. In this case, those might include:

- "What is this drug intended to do?"
- "*How* will we know if it's working for me?"
- "*When* will we know if it's working for me?"
- "What big problems should I be watching for, and what do I do if they occur?"

It's hard to be a successful CEO without good information. A logical question to ask is whether individuals are getting this kind of information from their doctors.

Who Knows?

In one study, doctors agreed to be recorded during patient visits as they prescribed drugs new to those individuals. Knowing that they were being recorded, doctors presumably were on their best behavior. Here is the percent of time that the doctors gave people the following critical pieces of information:

- reason for taking the drug: 87%
- name of the drug: 74%
- how often to take it: 68%
- how much to take each time: 55%
- side effects: 35%
- how long to keep taking the drug: 34%[144]

Assume that the doctors studied were all equally likely to perform at the above levels with every individual. The odds that any given person was told all six pieces of information are less than 3%.[145] The problem with that result is that people taking the drugs need to know all of these things.

Consider one of the higher percentages listed above: doctors told people the name of the drug 74% of the time. What difference does it make that they didn't tell everyone? Think about adverse drug events, discussed in Chapter One.

Who is present 100% of the time when a drug is being taken? It's not the doctors. It's the patients. How can they help prevent adverse drug events *that can kill them* if they aren't even told the name of the drug they are supposed to be getting? A quarter of the people weren't told.

If you aren't told the reason for taking the drug, the case with 13% of the individuals in this study:

- How could you have taken part in deciding whether to start taking it in the first place?
- How can you play an active role in figuring out if the drug's benefits outweigh any side effects?
- How do you take responsibility for managing the condition the drug is intended to treat?
- How likely are you to keep taking it?

Clearly, the necessary conversations are not happening. If health care were focused on you, a lot more attention would go into helping you figure out which of those four boxes you fall into, and advising you accordingly.

Connect the Docs

Curious about why doctors don't talk about side effects more often? The following experience suggests one reason. A Harvard Medical School student wondered why his professor so enthusiastically promoted cholesterol drugs, "and seemed to belittle a student who asked about side effects."[146]

It turned out that "The professor was not only a full-time member of the Harvard Medical faculty, but a paid consultant to 10 drug companies, including five makers of cholesterol treatments."[147]

Ties between doctors and manufacturers are common, and concern about them is increasing: "Federal health officials and prosecutors, frustrated that they have been unable to stop illegal kickbacks to doctors from drug and device companies, are investigating doctors who take money for using these products."[148]

"The move against doctors is part of a diverse campaign to curb industry marketing tactics that enrich doctors but increase health care costs and sometimes endanger patients."[149]

Doctors surveyed, by the way, believe that individuals should turn to them as the best source of quality information about drugs.[150]

Making the situation worse, "When patients feel they might be having an adverse drug effect, doctors will very often dismiss their concerns."[151] "'Physicians seem to commonly dismiss the possibility of a connection . . . even for the best-reported adverse effects of the most widely prescribed class of drugs.'"[152]

"Your bones are thinning."

After that first DEXAscan, I had two more over the next five years. By this time, I had switched to a new primary care physician, Dr. Wall.[153] She had been written up as one of the best family care practitioners in the state. She is intelligent, hard working, and thoughtful. Yet here is the entire communication I received — via recorded message — after the last DEXAscan: "Your bones are thinning. You need to start taking Drug A, [dosage and frequency]."

That was the same drug I had taken a few years earlier, with terrible side effects. I called her office and eventually connected with someone who was willing to answer questions, although I did not manage to get a live conversation with Dr. Wall herself.

"I need more information than I received in the voice mail I got about the DEXAscan I just had."

"It says here that your bones are thinning. You need to start taking Drug A."

"Yes, I got that message. I need some other information. For starters, what is the diagnosis? Do I have osteoporosis? Or is the diagnosis still osteopenia?" (Osteopenia is often, but not necessarily, a precursor to osteoporosis, which is a serious condition that can lead to bone fractures and other potentially disabling outcomes.)

"You have osteopenia."

"Okay. Good. And what are the actual test results?"

"Your bones are thinning, and you need to take Drug A."

"What I mean is, what are the numbers given in the report of the test?"

"I don't know. I'd have to find the report."

"Okay. I'll wait."

"Well, I might not be able to do that . . . I don't know if that's in your chart."

"Okay, I'll wait while you look."

"Well, hold on."

"Okay, thank you."

After a long wait, she read off a series of numbers. Among these was, "It says T is -2.1."

"Okay, and how does that compare to the last time I had the test?"

"I don't know."

"Could you look it up?"

"I don't know if we have that information."

"Yes, you do. Dr. Wall ordered the previous DEXAscan three and a half years ago. You have the results from that test. I'd like to know what the numbers are from that test so I can see how much they've changed in three and a half years."

After a longer wait, she read off the numbers, including, "T is -1.7."

"Thank you. What other treatment options are there? I cannot take Drug A. It was prescribed for me years ago and I experienced severe side effects. What other options do I have?"

"There isn't anything else. The only way to treat this is with one of these drugs, and they're all the same. Your bones are thinning and you have to start taking Drug A, [dosage, frequency]."

I ended the call, exasperated that there had been no discussion with me about options for a workable treatment plan — just an order for a drug that I knew I couldn't take. Experiences like mine are common. One study concluded that patients had a voice in treatment decisions only 9% of the time.[154]

Mushroom Treatment

It may feel to you as if the treatment you're getting most consistently regarding the course of action prescribed for you is the "mushroom treatment" — kept in the dark and fed manure.

The balance of this chapter provides details behind some of the information summarized above.

Coin Toss

The percentage of people who benefit from a treatment varies. For some treatments, it might be as high as 80%. For some, it might be as low as 30%. On average, it appears to be roughly 50%.[155]

For example, one drug company's press release announced that up to 30% of patients saw their pain reduced by half as a result of taking their drug, compared to 15% of patients who improved that much while taking a placebo[156] (pills that don't have any actual drug in them, commonly called "sugar pills"). Those numbers seem to imply that only 15 people out of 100 get significant benefits that they wouldn't get without the drug.

Before you page through the endnotes to find out which drug it is, note that it doesn't matter — the story would be very similar for many drugs, for many kinds of surgery, and for many other treatments as well. Here is another example: a new drug "normalized glucose levels in 51 percent of those who took it, compared with 30 percent in the placebo group."[157]

Here is how one writer summarized the data: "Difficult risk-benefit questions surround most drugs. . . . One dirty little secret of modern medicine is that many drugs work only in a minority of people."[158]

When a doctor orders a treatment for you, she doesn't typically have any idea if you're one of the roughly half who will be helped or one of the half who won't. She typically doesn't tell you that there's a good chance the treatment won't help you at all.

Success rates and side effects for surgery appear similar to those for drugs. As one example, the Blue Cross Blue Shield Technology Evaluation Center concluded that a particular kind of back surgery was successful 57% to 64% of the time.[159] Another analysis, published in a journal for bone surgeons, pegs it at 64%.[160]

There are side effects to surgery as well. For instance, according to Dr. Nortin Hadler of the University of North Carolina, coronary bypass surgery carries a 1-2% risk of death during the surgery, and up to a 40% chance of permanent mental decline.[161]

One Percent

When a drug is prescribed for you, do you have any idea what it is supposed to do and how much it is supposed to help you? For example, if the doctor says that you are at risk for a stroke and that taking this drug reduces that risk by half, does that mean:

- Out of 100 people at risk for a stroke, 100 will end up having a stroke without taking this medicine or something similar; with the medicine, only 50 of 100 will have a stroke?
- Out of 100 people at risk for a stroke, 2 will end up having a stroke without taking this medicine or something similar; with the medicine, only 1 out of 100 will have a stroke?

These both represent a 50% reduction in stroke risk.

The second of the above examples is more representative — one person in a hundred may benefit from a drug taken to forestall complications of a chronic condition.[162] For one diabetes drug, which had sales of $2.6 billion in one year, an almost infinite number of people would have to take the drug for one person to see a reduction in the consequences of diabetes.[163]

If the only boxes on the chart were the ones on the right — if there were no downsides to drugs — then one might be less concerned about numbers like this. But side effects abound, putting a lot of people in one of the boxes on the left-hand side of the chart.

A Hundred Pounds

To illustrate that side effects are a big part of the picture, this section provides more detail for one side effect: weight gain.

In talking about one class of drugs, The National Institutes of Health said, "Concerns have emerged in recent years that some of the newer medicines . . . can cause extreme weight gain, worsen cholesterol and lead to diabetes."[164]

Other researchers at well-respected medical centers echo these concerns. For example, an article reporting on an interview with the Director of the Johns Hopkins Weight Management Center noted, "Weight gain can range from a few pounds to more than a hundred pounds. . . . This excess weight is dangerous because it can cause or worsen problems like high blood pressure, other cardiovascular conditions, diabetes, high blood cholesterol, and osteoarthritis."[165]

A WebMD article noted, "Certain prescription drugs . . . can cause weight gain — sometimes 10 pounds a month. . . . Experts estimate the list [of prescription drugs that can cause weight gain] includes more than 50 common medications. . . . Medication-associated weight gain can be modest — or as much as 30 pounds over several months."[166]

A Mayo Clinic researcher commented, "Many physicians considered a drug's weight gain side effect to be a necessary evil . . . or assumed that only weight gains of 100 pounds or more were worrisome. But drugs that lead people to put on just 10 or 20 pounds a year, if taken for many years, can add up to big problems over time."[167]

Weight gain is only a problem if it's more than *a hundred pounds*? Doctors routinely tell patients that *losing* just 5-10% of their body weight can result in huge health improvements.[168] For someone who weighs 200 pounds, that's 10-20 pounds. It is surprising that many doctors have dismissed as unimportant *gaining* five to ten times as much weight.

One woman whose diabetes drug led to a 70-pound weight gain said, "I've been overweight my entire life. The last thing I needed was to gain more."[169] But the doctor who prescribed the drug apparently never discussed this side effect with her. He had five years to do it — that's how long he kept her on the drug.

The most likely explanation is that the doctor is accustomed to considering only the actions he takes (prescribe the drug). The doctor is not accustomed to considering the patient's resulting experience, which in this case almost certainly included a worsening of her health.

When she changed to a new doctor, he changed her drugs. Over the course of the next year, she lost the 70 pounds. For many people, however, once weight is gained, it is never lost.[170]

In fact, given the volume of drugs prescribed in the U.S., one wonders what percent of the obesity epidemic is a direct result of drug prescriptions. Half of the adults in the U.S. report taking prescription medicine daily.[171]

Be Wary

In an article titled, "Be Wary of Narcotics to Treat Back Pain," *Consumer Reports* notes that such drugs often don't do much to help the pain.

At the same time, "Clinical trials have shown that about half of the people who take them suffer adverse effects such as drowsiness, respiratory depression, and gastrointestinal symptoms such as constipation, reflux, heartburn, cramping, nausea, and vomiting. Moreover, other adverse effects of opioids include a paradoxical increase in pain sensitivity, reduced testosterone levels, and erectile dysfunction. . . . The side effects often outweigh the benefits."[172]

Despite the above, more people are being prescribed these drugs — a trend the author attributes to extensive marketing.[173]

My Way or the Highway

Imagine a marriage in which one partner's stance is, "I'll tell you what to do, and if you disagree with me about anything, you can leave. We'll get a divorce." Does that sound like a relationship that would encourage you to engage, ask questions, and explore the pros and cons of different choices?

Now consider how one doctor described the relationship between doctors and patients: "The physician-patient compact basically states that a doctor will care for a patient in exchange for compensation and that the patient will heed the doctor's advice. Patients who disagree with their physicians . . . are free to go elsewhere."[174] Does *that* sound like a relationship that would encourage you to engage, ask questions, and explore the pros and cons of different choices?

Health care professionals and policy makers want you to take more responsibility for your health. Part of what they often mean is that they want you to do as you are told. In other words, you are expected to comply with orders given by someone who may focus more on ordering treatments than on what happens to you as a result.

Whose Choice?

Doctors get incensed whenever insurance companies make decisions about what care they can deliver (or, to be more precise, what care the insurance company will pay for). That's understandable; none of us likes to have someone breathing down our neck, second-guessing everything we do. Doctors want to rely on their judgment and make the decisions.

Two issues with that stance are worth noting. The first issue is that only about 20-25% of treatments actually have enough facts backing them up to allow one to say for sure whether the treatment genuinely helps.[175] "Treatments are based largely on rules and traditions, not scientific evidence."[176]

The second issue is that choices are not always clear-cut. As with everything that you purchase, each option may have some features you really like that other options don't have — and each option may have its own drawbacks. That's where values and priorities come in. The question is *whose*.

For example, if you ask surgeons if you should have surgery, it's not terribly surprising that they say yes a large percentage of the time. Performing surgery is what they do. That doesn't mean that surgery is necessarily the best choice for you. Researchers at Dartmouth did some very clever studies which showed that it is usually the *doctor's* values and priorities that get applied — not those of the person who has to live with the results.[177]

When science shows that the outcomes of two treatments are similar, it would make sense for people to be told the pros and cons of each option and then to decide which one to have, based on their own sense of priorities.[178] However, the patients' preferences often do not guide the decisions in these cases.

When individuals have complete information, they make choices that are very different from those that doctors make.[179] They choose less invasive, less aggressive treatments as much as *60% more often* than do people who aren't given that information and who instead follow their doctors' lead.[180]

Here is an example of what happens when people have information about outcomes. Medicare commissioned a study to decide whether to pay for "lung volume reduction surgery" for emphysema.[181] The idea is that with the diseased part of the lung removed, the remaining part of the lung will work better. Before the study was done, people took it for granted that the surgery was a life-saving miracle. However, here's what the study showed:

- Eight percent of patients died as a result of the surgery.
- Most people who had the surgery didn't survive any longer than the people who didn't have it.
- A higher percentage of people who had the surgery ended up back in the hospital or in a nursing home in the months following the surgery, compared to similar patients who didn't have the surgery.
- A small group of people did live longer.[182]

Because the lung surgery did help a small subset of the population, Medicare decided to publicize the study and pay for the surgery. The economists were frantic. They thought that "tens of thousands"[183] of people would go under the knife, at $50,000 each. They thought this treatment would break the bank. What actually happened? In the first 21 months only 458 people had the surgery.[184]

The barriers to adopting patient aids for decision-making (such as charts comparing options) lie largely with doctors. For instance, one study notes that one barrier is the need to prove to practitioners that such aids will help them by "saving time, avoiding repetition [having to explain things to patients], not requiring extra calls from patients, potentially decreasing liability, and potentially reducing wait-list pressures."[185]

Notice that that nowhere in the list of benefits doctors seek is assurance that they are providing the treatment that best meets patients' priorities and needs.

CHAPTER SIX

"Keep Away"

It is not always obvious what is wrong with you when you fall ill. Getting a diagnosis can be time-consuming and nerve-wracking. One of the more upsetting aspects of the experience is that it is often very hard to find out what is happening as the days and weeks scroll by and the doctors are getting your test results and perhaps talking with each other — but not talking with you.

Playground

In the children's ball game "Keep Away," all the people in a circle around the person in the center do their best to keep the ball away from him or her.[186] When you are sick, it can feel as if the professionals are playing "Keep Away" — with you in the center.

Here's what one expert observed: "Healthcare systems have always transferred uncertainty and risk to the patient. Managers, doctors and nurses are in control; they have certainty, it is the patient who usually does not know what is going to happen, or when or why. The risk is taken by the patient rather than the doctor."[187]

The consequences to you of playing an involuntary game of "Keep Away" are both subtle and debilitating. At the very least, "Keep Away" saps your energy, demoralizes and degrades you, and can easily induce high stress levels — all things that can create serious health problems all by themselves. An example of "Keep Away" in the process of getting a diagnosis of a potentially serious condition follows.

Endometrial Cancer

Two and a half years after my last menstrual period, I had another one. That seemed unusual, so I called my doctor's office to ask, "Is this okay, or does this require some kind of attention?" Later in the day, I got a message saying that I should come in. When I called back and was transferred to the scheduling person, she told me that the first available appointment was two weeks away.

I asked if Dr. Wall understood when she said that I should come in that it meant waiting two weeks. The scheduler didn't know. I said that I would like to know if the doctor understood the lead time I would be given, or if my situation meant I should be given an "urgent" slot on her schedule. After several phone calls back and forth, I was still unable to get an answer to this question. Eventually, at my insistence, the scheduler ungraciously agreed that I could come in sooner.

Notice here that, as the patient, I had no idea what the doctor was thinking — is this urgent or is this routine? Thus I had no idea how aggressively to push for an appointment, rearrange my own work commitments to be able to get to the doctor's office on short notice, and so forth. This "not knowing" is nerve-wracking all by itself.

Fault

When I saw the doctor, she explained that it was necessary to rule out endometrial cancer. She looked at her records and said disapprovingly, "You're overdue for a Pap smear."

I replied, "No, I am not. It hasn't even been two years, and you told me that I did not need to have the next one for three years."

"Well," she replied, "I said that you *could* wait two or three years. I didn't say that you *had* to wait."

"You told me that there was no reason for me to come in sooner," I reminded her. I found it annoying — and a routine experience — to immediately be told that I had done something wrong, when I had simply followed her advice.

It unsettled me — was this conversation about whose fault it was if I had cancer? I just needed a diagnosis. I didn't need finger-pointing. Why was this the starting point she chose?

Time Line

She laid out a series of diagnostic tests to be done, in sequence:

- blood tests to check hormone levels
- pelvic ultrasound to see the lining of the uterus
- gynecological exam including a pap smear
- either an endometrial biopsy or a D&C (dilation & curettage); the D&C would be chosen if the endometrium appeared thick in the ultrasound

I asked how long this sequence of procedures would take to complete. She said that it would be at least six weeks. I asked if we could schedule all of the steps now, to reduce the lead time involved in waiting for appointments.

She said no, that it was necessary to know the results of each step before one knew for certain what the next step should be. I commented that I was concerned about taking so long to get a diagnosis; if I had cancer, it seemed to me that it would be better to know as quickly as possible.

"Oh, you have time," she said dismissively.

The ultrasound was scheduled for a few days later. At the imaging center, they told me that if I hadn't heard from my doctor after four days, I should call her. I did not hear from her, and was able to get through to her on the fifth day. She told me that I should now schedule the pelvic exam and Pap smear. The first open appointment on her calendar was five days later.

Stages

With the above information, I called a health care help line to which I had access. Their marketing materials encouraged people to call them for advice about medical conditions and treatments. I had one question: how fast does endometrial cancer develop?

As I understood it, the severity of cancer is indicated by its stage. In Stage I, for instance, the cancer is small. It is contained in one area, and often can be easily treated. In Stage IV, the cancer has spread, or has other characteristics which mean that the prognosis is grim.[188]

I wanted to know how quickly endometrial cancer progresses from Stage I to Stage II to Stage III to Stage IV. I was concerned about the weeks that would go by before I even had a diagnosis.

After doing some research, the help line nurse called me back: she had been unable to find any information about how fast endometrial cancer progresses. I was incredulous. It seemed to me that this was the one crucial piece of information a patient needed to know in thinking about the timeline for testing and treatment.

She asked me if I trusted my doctor. "She's a good doctor," I said.

"Well," the help line nurse said, "then you should just go with what she's telling you."

"You understand that what you're telling me is not logic-based?" I asked. "If you can't find this information and your organization's entire job is research, why would you think that my primary care doctor, whose entire job is seeing patients, would have access to better information than you do about a condition she probably doesn't see very often?"

She had no answer.

Seventeen Days

I went for the gynecological exam. Dr. Wall told me that it would take a minimum of ten days to get the Pap smear results. Then it would take her some time to consult with Dr. Green,[189] the specialist she recommended.

She would ask him whether he thought an endometrial biopsy was best or if a D&C would be needed instead. I asked her if she couldn't ask him that question now. She said no, he would want to know what the Pap smear results were before he said anything.

The clock was ticking.

I waited anxiously for ten days. Then I started calling the service that provides test results for my doctor's office. Here's how it works: someone in the doctor's office records a message on this service providing the test results. Then the doctor's office calls you and leaves a voice mail telling you that you have test results available at a 1-800 number. Then you retrieve the message via the password-protected message service.

In this way, the doctor's office knows they aren't violating your privacy by leaving a message with medical information in it on an answering machine that perhaps many other people have access to. I hadn't gotten any message from the doctor's office, but I didn't want to make a pest of myself and keep asking them for my Pap smear results, so instead I just called the message number every day to see if any results for me had been recorded. There weren't any.

Seventeen days after the Pap smear, I still hadn't heard from the doctor's office. After a series of calls asking for information, here is the conversation I had with one of her staff:

"She called you three days after the Pap smear to give you the results. You never called her back."

"What?! I never got any message!"

"She called you. You didn't call back."

I was working very hard trying to follow this conversation. Here's what I didn't understand:

- No one picks up my voice mail at work but me, and there was no message from the doctor. My husband doesn't answer the phone at home. Everything goes to the answering machine, and there was no message. So this did not happen.
- They have a process for reporting test results. It involves leaving a message to call the 1-800 number. And even if I somehow missed the message, I'd been checking the test results message line, and there was never any message there for me. So that did not happen.
- It had been 17 days; she was saying they had called two weeks ago and hadn't heard back from me. Were they never going to try to call me again? They think that I may have cancer, but they're not going to try to get in touch with me to tell me what to do next?
- Dr. Wall had told me that it always takes at least 10 days to get Pap smear results. Her motivation in giving me this protracted timeline was probably to buy herself time to have a chance to talk with Dr. Green. But wouldn't you think that she

would know that I'd want to hear the Pap smear results as soon as they were available? After all, we were talking about cancer!

I said, "Look, I never got a message. I'm on the phone now. Can I talk with her?" Predictably, Dr. Wall wasn't available. I was promised a call back. After a while, I got a call saying, "Dr. Wall says that you can make an appointment to see Dr. Green or any other ob/gyn and have either an endometrial biopsy or a D&C."

Making Sense

The problems I had with this message are hard to count:

- If the tests weren't going to clarify the next step needed, why did I spend four weeks having them and waiting for the results?
- Dr. Wall had said that she would consult with Dr. Green and let me know what his recommendation was. Now I was supposed to just pick somebody at random to go see? What was I supposed to tell that doctor? That I'd had a number of tests but didn't know most of the results and didn't have any paperwork reporting on any of them?
- Was I supposed to flip a coin? Heads, ask for an endometrial biopsy; tails, ask for a D&C? Or was the doctor supposed to flip a coin? What were the decision criteria supposed to be?
- Why didn't I have a better understanding of what was going on?

I said, "What does that mean? Did Dr. Wall talk to Dr. Green? If so, what did he say? If not, is she going to? She told me that she would talk with him and let me know what he recommended."

"It says here that you can make an appointment to see Dr. Green or any other ob/gyn and have either an endometrial biopsy or a D&C."

"Yes, I heard that, but that doesn't make any sense! Please, I need to talk to Dr. Wall. This is very upsetting. I don't understand what is happening."

"Dr. Wall has left the office for the day and won't be back for another two days. I'll leave her a message."

"Another two days!" It felt very much like "Keep Away."

"Yes, two days."

"Well, can you at least tell me what the result of the Pap smear was?"

"Oh. It was negative."

I have no record of ever hearing the results of the blood tests. Despite asking at least twice, I never received a copy of the results for my records. I didn't even know exactly what the tests were. It had now been almost five weeks since I had had the unexpected period.

Doctor's Practice

Two days later the doctor called. I explained all of the above. She said, "I didn't call you! I never left you a message. I don't know why they told you that. Who told you that?"

I said, "I don't know. It was a very upsetting conversation. I didn't catch her name — if she even gave it to me. They usually say something like, 'I'm calling from Dr. Wall's office.'"

She said, "You should keep a record of who you talk to in my office. There's nothing I can do about it if I don't know who you talked to."

It did not occur to me until later to realize I should have told her to look at the signature on the pink message slip she had in her hand asking her to call me. That's the person I talked with. I was disheartened again that gaps in her practice were being framed as my failures.

"There's no note in the file to say I called you. I hadn't gotten around to talking to Dr. Green yet, so I hadn't called you. After all, it wasn't an emergency. I told you it wasn't urgent. So it was just sitting on my desk waiting until I had a chance to get to it."

Now I was thinking, "How is it supposed to improve my health for me to go for an extra three weeks in limbo, not knowing if it looks like I have cancer or not? And if I have cancer, letting it continue to progress? What is the definition of urgent? Urgent to whom?"

"But what did Dr. Green say? You were going to talk with him and he was going to say whether an endometrial biopsy was next or a D&C, so that I knew what kind of appointment to schedule."

"Oh, he would want to examine you himself. He couldn't really say without examining you. So if you want to see him, you should make an appointment with him. He'll examine you, and then he'll decide what to schedule next. Or you can choose someone else to go to."

I said, "I don't have any basis for choosing anybody, so if you say he's good, I'll go to him. But this sounds like more lead time — lead time to get an appointment with him, then lead time before the next procedure."

"This is what you need to do."

Invalid Test Results

I made an appointment with Dr. Green. After he examined me, he performed an endometrial biopsy. He told me to make an appointment for a follow-up ultrasound six weeks after the first one, and then to make an appointment to come back and see him to hear the results of the biopsy and the ultrasound.

He also told me that the report on the first ultrasound omitted the one critical piece of information he needed, the thickness of the endometrial lining. He mentioned casually that he'd call over sometime and get the testing site to tell him that if they could. But I never heard anything back about it.

I found this very upsetting: if the whole point of the ultrasound was to provide this piece of information, and that was supposed to inform his choice of the next procedure, why wasn't it important to get that information before proceeding? It seemed that the ultrasound had served no purpose at all.

Two Months

I had made a great deal of effort to rearrange my commitments at work to go to various appointments and have all the tests and procedures. All that time and effort didn't seem to have gotten me any further along in understanding what was happening.

It wasn't just a question of the time from work, of course. It was the mental and emotional wear and tear as well. I wondered:

- Why hadn't Dr. Green called to try to get the information about the ultrasound before my appointment — or while I was there — if that was the one critical piece of information he needed to inform his actions?
- Why did he insist that every test result required an office visit to impart?
- Why did I have to wait until the results of the ultrasound were available to hear the results of the biopsy?
- Why did I repeatedly feel that I didn't know what was going on?

Two months to the day after I had first contacted Dr. Wall, I was back in Dr. Green's office. For almost two months, I had been laboring under the weight of the possibility that I might have cancer, and that day by day, it might be progressing at an unknown speed — and ultimately, result in my death.

I sat in Dr. Green's office, waiting for him to speak. "You don't have cancer," he said offhandedly. "We don't know why, but sometimes women just have another period after you'd think they wouldn't. That seems to be what happened here. You don't need any follow-up unless you have further bleeding or other symptoms."

Stress

And that was the end of it. Two months of extreme distress — caused not by any medical condition, but by being kept off balance and uninformed.

The distress was caused by being treated by two good doctors as if how I felt about what was going on wasn't part of the equation. If I had thought that they were incompetent, it would actually have been easier: they would just have been doctors to avoid. But they are both intelligent, capable, well-regarded professionals.

That fact just highlights the pervasive dysfunction of the health care system. The biggest issues are not typically about individual doctors being incompetent. The biggest issues are about the entire framework of health care being skewed, off-kilter, focused incorrectly — missing the point that health care should be about enhancing your well-being.

Silent Messages

When a patient is treated as I was, what are the silent messages she hears?

- "We have an approach to getting a diagnosis. We are comfortable that it makes sense. How you feel or what you need to know to feel comfortable with that approach is not important. Just do as we say."
- "We will tell you that the length of time we will take to arrive at a diagnosis doesn't create any problems for you, but we won't give you any information to support that view."
- "We will create artificial lead-times to give ourselves some leeway."
- "Telling you your test results is not a priority. It may be weeks after we've had the results before we tell you what they were — if we ever tell you."
- "Sometimes test results are clearly incomplete or wrong, but it's not a priority to get that sorted out. There's also no need for us to explain to you why we feel that it's not important to get meaningful results from tests that we told you it was essential to have."
- "We won't give you the actual reports of your test results. Those are for us."
- "If you have a problem, it must be your fault."

Intelligent Consumer

Now consider that picture in light of the idea that we are all supposed to be intelligent health care consumers, making informed purchase decisions. First, we are supposed to decide what proposed actions to reject outright, and then decide where to have procedures done based on cost and quality data.

This idea becomes laughable when set up against the situation I faced. I had no way of knowing if all those tests — blood tests, two ultrasounds, a pelvic exam, a Pap smear, and an endometrial biopsy — were necessary or not.

They were all presented ahead of time as essential steps in the diagnostic process. However, each one in turn appeared to be dismissed as irrelevant or uninformative after the fact, and did not seem to influence what happened next. But I had no way to figure out up front if they were worth paying for.

"Keep Away."

CHAPTER SEVEN

Children's Table at Thanksgiving

Many doctors do not want to give you ready access to the information in your medical record. Studies show that they prefer to keep to themselves most of the important information, such as their notes and significant test results. Being out of the loop for essential information hampers your efforts to manage and improve your health.

Check Out

If you're like many people, you may not get basic information that your doctor has about you which *you* need in order to manage your health. For example, a Mayo Clinic study showed that when checking out of the hospital, only 42% of the patients even knew their diagnoses, and only 28% knew the names of the drugs they were taking.[190]

How could the 58% who didn't know their diagnoses tell the next doctor they saw their medical history? How could the 72% who didn't know the names of the drugs they were taking help prevent adverse drug events? You can't even be a successful bit player in your own health drama without having this kind of information. You certainly can't play a leading role.

Segregating the Children

Think about every family Thanksgiving dinner you've ever attended. Why is it traditional to seat the children at card tables — preferably in a different room — while the grown-ups eat in the dining room?

A common answer is that it allows the grown-ups to talk among themselves and say things that it is not appropriate for the children to hear.[191] If it were simply a matter of space, one could put both adults and children in each room.

It's not about space.

Seating You at the Children's Table

Today, most information about your medical care is probably handwritten in file folders all over town — or all over the country, if you've moved around. There's a lot of discussion about putting it on computers in the form of EMR (Electronic Medical Records) or EHR (Electronic Health Records).

The idea is that if your information were in electronic form, doctors and hospitals would be able to provide you with much better care. As an example, one doctor would be able to see the results of tests that another doctor had already run. Then there would be no delays or duplication resulting from the second doctor's ordering a test you had already had. Other benefits abound.

Wouldn't it be great if you could have access to all your medical records online, similar to the way you have access to records of your online purchases through Amazon.com? You might consider this idea to be a no-brainer. The health care profession doesn't.

One study reported, "Clinicians expressed concern about problems that could arise if patients have access to clinical notes. They believed that they needed to be frank in documenting patient problems and conditions but were concerned that the language and content of their notes could upset patients if they were able to read them."[192]

On a similar note, "The medical record for so many years has been the private domain of the physician, and the notion of using it as a shared document is relatively new."[193]

One doctor said, "I would certainly dumb down what I said in the record so they would be able to understand it — I would have to. I would be now dictating a note to the patient rather than a note to myself if I know that they have access to the record right now."[194]

The record that everyone agrees *you* should have ready access to is a PHR (Personal Health Record.) This is a record *you* keep, and it contains information about "daily symptoms, over-the-counter medicines taken, personal exercise programs, special diets, or data from home monitoring devices."[195]

It can be very useful to record that information. However, when you are told that that is all you can have ready access to, it feels like being seated at the children's table at Thanksgiving. The traditional, hard-core medical information — test results and results of physical exams the doctors perform, for instance — would be in the EHR or EMR, the province of doctors.

In some cases, individuals may be given limited access to some items in their EHR/EMR, but be blocked from seeing some of the information such as the doctor's notes. In California, it's illegal for you to get some of your medical test results electronically. Ever. Even if you sign something saying that you want them.[196] Elsewhere, there may not be state laws, but doctors often take a similar stance.

You have a legal right in all 50 states to see the entire content of your medical record.[197] (In some cases there may be exceptions related to mental illness or alcohol or substance abuse.) But often you must jump through hoops. Either you have to go to the doctor's office to see your record, or you typically must put the request in writing and either hand deliver it or send it by mail — not by e-mail.

Many care providers require that you fill out a particular form to request a copy of your records. Often, these forms are not available on line, so just getting the blank form takes some effort. There is no charge for you to *see* your record. However, if you want a copy to keep, you may have to pay a fee, such as a dollar a page. It may take thirty days for you to receive your records.

Those records may be constantly changing. More information is added every time you visit the doctor. It would be quite tedious to go through the above process after every doctor's visit or other interaction with the health care system.

Thus, it takes much more effort for you to see your medical records than it does to see other information that relates to you. For example, many health insurance companies provide online access to claim and benefit information that you can access at no charge virtually anytime.

It's very common for medical records — paper or electronic — to have mistakes in them that only you would realize. In one study surveying people who did have access to their medical records, 25% reported finding errors.[198] Making your medical records hard for you to access increases the probability of misdiagnoses, medical errors, and adverse drug events — all of which can kill you.

Sunday, 2:00 a.m.

One doctor commented, "I think it would be — at best an inconvenience for me that I would no longer feel comfortable putting down: 'There's a distant possibility of a brain tumor. If the headaches are still going on two weeks from now, let's get a CT scan.'"[199]

Play that example out. Suppose that you have not seen your medical records, or even more dangerous, that the doctor has started keeping a "second set of books," so to speak: keeping notes about you that she doesn't put into your official medical record and doesn't tell you about. Then suppose that you end up in the emergency room at 2:00 a.m. on Sunday.

If your doctor thinks there's even a slight chance that you might have a brain tumor, your ignorance of that fact doesn't help you get better care. It endangers your life. Misdiagnosis rates in the ER run as high as 40%.[200] The less information you can contribute, the greater the chance that harried ER staff will miss something important.

The doctor isn't with you 24 hours a day, 7 days a week, to provide this information. The only person there all the time is you. Keeping individuals in the dark reflects a belief that only doctors need to understand what is going on in the individual's body. But they are not living in it. They are not the ones experiencing the symptoms, or the side effects of treatment.

One independent study noted, "Patients have little access to information and knowledge that can help them participate in, let alone guide, their own care. . . . At a minimum, they need access to information from their providers' EHRs — their own diagnoses, medications, allergies, lab test results, visit summaries, and other findings over time."[201]

It is very rare that your health will be better as a result of being prevented from having ready access to your own medical record. Being seated at the children's table does not serve you well.

Testing Patience

On a similar note, people typically cannot get their own medical test results as soon as they are available; they must wait until the doctor releases them. Why? Doctors argue that patients won't know how to interpret them and may be upset and confused.[202]

That view implies that people are less distressed by waiting than they are by getting the test results promptly from the testing service or from a staff member in the doctor's office. That is a questionable position, for two reasons.

First, most tests are done to rule out problems, and that's exactly what they do. Said another way, most of the results come back saying, "No, you don't have this disease."

By one calculation, for instance, 100-200 women get mammograms for every one diagnosed with cancer.[203] To make it simple, assume that one person has cancer for every one hundred who are tested. That means that 99 women out of 100 would be relieved, not upset or confused, when they got their results.[204]

Second, research shows that uncertainty all by itself is harmful to people. Even the one person with cancer would be better off knowing as soon as possible, rather than waiting for an extended period for the doctor to have a chance to call.

A Harvard professor reports that research shows that people "feel worse when something bad *might* occur than when something bad *will* occur. . . . Human beings find uncertainty more painful than the things they're uncertain about."[205]

He goes on to say, "Why would we prefer to know the worst than to suspect it? Because when we get bad news we weep for a while, and then get busy making the best of it. . . . But we can't come to terms with circumstances whose terms we don't know yet. An uncertain future leaves us stranded in an unhappy present with nothing to do but wait."[206]

Here's how a *New York Times* article described the experience of one woman waiting for cancer test results, which her doctor had promised to get to her in the two days before he left on an extended vacation: "Freddie Odlum spent two terrible days waiting by the phone for her doctor to call. . . . 'All those clichés when someone is facing a terminal diagnosis are used because they are true,' she said. 'Racing pulse, dry mouth, total self-preoccupation with what-ifs to the point that real life doesn't exist, willing the phone to ring.'"[207]

When she hadn't heard anything on the first day, she left messages begging him to call her before he left town. The second day, she waited, "'jumping at every noise, not letting anyone use the phone, imagining every scenario.' Her doctor left for his vacation. He never called, not even when he returned."[208]

An article about women being tested for breast cancer carried the headline, "Study Equates Stress of Cancer and of Wait for Biopsy Results."[209] Fifty-eight percent of the women were still waiting for their test results after five days. They had blood levels of a stress hormone, cortisol, *identical* to those of women who had learned that they had cancer.

The article goes on to say, "Cortisol levels can influence wound healing and immune response, raising a woman's potential health risks. . . . And the stress and anxiety of waiting also affects the quality of life of a woman and her family and her ability to function well at work."[210]

Other research shows "Psychological stress can take a physical toll on many body systems, causing, for instance:

- increased blood pressure
- increased heart rate
- muscle aches
- digestive problems
- weakened immune system
- skin disorders
- allergies, asthma
- increased sensitivity to pain"[211]

One news article reported, "Studies suggest that high levels of stress can lead to obesity and trigger a raft of diseases — from heart attacks to ulcers. These and other stress-related diseases sicken millions of people each year in the USA, says brain researcher Bruce McEwen at the Rockefeller University in New York."[212]

The article continues, "Up to 90% of the doctor visits in the USA may be triggered by a stress-related illness, says the Centers for Disease Control and Prevention. . . . New research suggests that over-the-top stress can go beyond the temporary increase in blood pressure to actually injure cells of the body. That injury may accelerate the aging process, leaving people prone to a laundry list of diseases."[213]

Virtually all health care providers are interested in enhancing people's health rather than in damaging it. Interacting with patients in ways deliberately designed to *reduce* their stress levels — rather than unthinkingly *increase* them — might be one of the best ways they could contribute to their patients' health.

Since not knowing the results of medical tests causes high stress levels, and high stress levels damage health, the most effective way to have test results enhance rather than damage people's health is to provide them as quickly as possible. That generally means not making people wait for the doctor to call them. Results typically could be provided more quickly by other staff members or through an automated system.

Black Hole

You might wait forever if you wait for the doctor to tell you your test results. One study revealed that doctors themselves say that they report normal test results to patients only 14% - 37% of the time. They say that they report abnormal test results to patients 55% to 71% of the time.[214]

Here's what one doctor said in defense of physicians who don't inform patients of their test results: "The biggest mistake we see when we see these things not dealt with is when the doctor knows the patient has an appointment in a month and plans to deal with it then, and then the patient doesn't show up."[215]

Notice the implication that it is the *patients'* fault that the doctor doesn't notify them of test results. Notice also that waiting a month to tell people their test results is considered completely fine — by the doctor.

"And in many cases, doctors may choose not to call patients 'because we know that they know we know what's going on, and they trust us, so we don't call unless it's necessary,' he says. 'We have found when we call patients about lab results, they give us better patient satisfaction scores. But we don't want to call with information that could confuse them, give them more information than they need for some minor change. You can create anxiety. If the result is expected or not relevant, we don't call.'"[216]

Notice here that the patients have voted in favor of getting their test results; that's what the patient satisfaction survey results indicate. Notice that the doctor, *knowing what the patients prefer*, has decided that doing the opposite is best for them.

If you *never* hear the test results from the doctor, what does that do to your stress levels? And can you assume that if you don't hear, it means everything is okay? No, that's a potentially deadly assumption. Your results indicating a serious problem simply may have been filed away by accident. One study showed that "1% to 10% of clinically important abnormal test results are missed by providers, with potential adverse consequences for patients' health."[217]

Another study concluded that doctors fail to report such results to patients on average 7% of the time. In some doctors' practices, patients are not informed of serious abnormal results in more than 20% of the cases.[218] Said another way, test results show that something is seriously wrong and needs prompt attention — and the doctor *never* tells you.

It certainly feels as if you're being relegated to the children's table, out of the loop for important information.

Sleeping Beauty

When would people be better off not getting test results, or not getting them promptly? The most likely answer is: when they have no idea what they are being tested for. Then they might have very little concern about the results. But that situation is not plausible because it means that people would be expected to undergo tests — potentially expensive, dangerous tests, or tests that require them to give up bodily fluids or tissue samples — without even knowing why.

If people are expected to be intelligent consumers of health care, they need to know why tests are being run. If they know what the test is for, then obviously they know what the potential outcomes are. For example, if they are being tested for diabetes, one possible outcome of the test is that they have diabetes.

So what would doctors have to believe to conclude that waiting for an appointment to hear your results, playing telephone tag, or never getting your test results at all is less upsetting to you than getting the results from another staff member or from the testing service — or via an automated process — as soon as they are available?

They would have to believe that you are in a state of suspended animation, that you have no thoughts or feelings at all until they interact with you — like Sleeping Beauty being dead to the world until the prince kisses her. That's not a description of a health care system that's about you. That's a description of a health care system that's about doctors.

Uninformed Consent

Ironically, informed consent forms provide another example of how hard it is for you to get important information. The forms are typically written without regard for anyone's ability to understand them.

"Almost half of Americans read at or below the eight-grade level."[219] Most informed consent forms are written about *three grade levels higher*.[220] In fact, 41% - 75% of patients in one study could not understand informed consent forms.[221]

Would you immediately realize that a "percutaneous endoscopic gastrostomy tube" is a feeding tube?[222] You're unlikely to find references to feeding tubes in informed consent forms; you're more likely to see the jargon.

Attempts to simplify the language are resisted, because informed consent forms are viewed as "legal tools."[223] Said another way, it's not about whether you understand what is going to be done to you when you undergo surgery or other major treatment — actions that could radically change — or end — your life. It's about making it harder for you to sue.

That's not individual-centric.

Understanding

Does it matter if you understand what's going on when you are involved with the health care system? Yes, it does. "Problems with communication between patients and health care providers can increase risk for injury or death for those who require medical care. . . . 'More serious adverse events are caused by communication problems than any other thing.'"[224]

"Experts agree that if the industry is to keep lowering the rate of medical errors and unsafe care, patients will have to monitor their own care and speak up when it appears that something's wrong. But if professional caregivers can't speak in a jargon-free manner — addressing the patient at their level of literacy or respect cultural differences — that's virtually impossible."[225]

Interestingly enough, the blame for this gap is placed in the lap of individuals. The title of a *USA Today* article is telling. *USA Today* does an exceptionally fine job of explaining complex ideas about the health care system in a way that is both accurate and easy to understand.

But even they, this time, fell prey to "blame the victim." One article is titled, "Patient Illiteracy Threatens Health Care."[226] Why not, "Health Care Kills People by Failing to Explain Clearly"? Why is it that the *patients* are at fault here?

People don't understand or remember much of what doctors tell them. "If you are a typical patient, you remember less than half of what your doctor tries to explain," regardless of your education or economic status.[227] Further, "almost half of the information that is remembered is incorrect."[228]

It is common for patients to experience "anxiety and distress"[229] during doctors' appointments, making it harder for them to remember what they are told. Research also shows that doctors typically provide information orally and in a disorganized way, making it unlikely that people will remember it. One study found that "with spoken medical instructions only 14% of the information was remembered correctly."[230]

A basic rule for any person or organization offering services to the public is that it's essential to provide people with what they need and/or want. It's curious that the health care system assumes that it's not at all necessary to provide people with what they need most if they are to take responsibility for their own health: clear and understandable information about what's going on in their own bodies.

It's worth noting that there are now entire businesses that thrive by getting paid to help patients decipher what they're told.[231]

Mushrooms as Decision-Makers

Two ways of thinking about the individual are on a collision course. The first was introduced in Chapter Five: "patients are mushrooms," kept in the dark. People are fed filtered and restricted information on somebody else's timeline.

The second, which was mentioned briefly in Chapter Six, is currently championed by people who write the checks for health care, such as employers. It is "if they have to pay more of the costs themselves, consumers will be intelligent decision-makers." The individual-as-mushroom and individual-as-decision-maker ideas are not consistent with each other.

If on one hand you're treated like someone without any intelligence who isn't even included in the discussion about what might be going on in your own body, you can't flip a switch and suddenly become an engaged and empowered consumer on the other. It's very hard to play the role of an oblivious baby about whom other people make all the decisions one minute and the role of a grown-up the next.

The mushroom approach may have worked for the Norman Rockwell doctor of the 1950s, but it doesn't fit today. Some health care professionals argue that "many people don't want to know — they still want the Norman Rockwell doctor."

That argument is like saying that no women should be permitted to go to college because some women aspire to be waitresses. While waitressing is a needed service, it doesn't require a college degree. Therefore, no women should be allowed to go to college.

No one would stand for such an argument today outside of health care. What does it mean? That everyone should be kept in the dark and hobbled in their efforts to improve their own health because if the information were available, not everyone would take advantage of it?

A general lament among health care experts is that individuals don't take a more active role in managing their own health. Given the discussion in this book so far, it is clear that one of the reasons people don't do so is that they are often subtly discouraged from meaningful involvement — at every step.

CHAPTER EIGHT

"I don't get no respect." "I can't get no satisfaction."

When a patient reports facts that don't square with the doctor's assumptions, it's often the facts that get discarded. To account for taking this approach, doctors sometimes assert that the patient is lying or mentally ill, or both. Furthermore, doctors often discount concerns of vital importance to patients, or fail to consider their perspective, leaving them feeling diminished.

The comedian Rodney Dangerfield could have been speaking for patients everywhere with his trademark lament, as could the Rolling Stones with the refrain of their famous rock song. Individuals' experiences of their own health are discounted and their voices often go unheard.

Thirteen Cotton Balls

In December of my second year of graduate school, I came down with an earache. It felt like an ice pick inside my skull. I went to the student health clinic. The specialist the university had on tap prescribed a decongestant that in my prior experience had caused serious side effects. I explained to him that I got extremely hyper on that drug and had been advised never to take it again.

He told me to take it anyway. I did, and ended up not sleeping for four days. I landed back in the student health clinic in a very agitated state. Of course, the doctor I saw on an emergency basis included in her discharge instructions that I should never take that drug again.

A few days later, I returned to the student health clinic to see the specialist yet again. I told him that I had been seen a few days earlier for a severe reaction to the decongestant and that he could find a record of that visit in my chart. However, he did not have my chart and made no move to ask for it. He again told me that I had to take the drug.

He also told me that I should pinch my nostrils shut and blow very hard to clear my ears. The next time I saw him, I told him that this maneuver was excruciatingly painful. He told me to do it anyway. In ways large and small, it became clear that he had little patience for my experience of my body and my illness.

Months went by. Although the "ice pick" pain had been relieved early on, I couldn't hear well because my ear was full of fluid, and I felt peculiar. It was now April. A dozen visits and five months of assorted drug therapies hadn't eliminated the fluid.

The doctor was clearly getting frustrated. He decided to slice my eardrum open to drain the fluid. After doing so, he told me that my problems were over, that he had suctioned out all the fluid, and that no more would accumulate.

I slept badly that night. I kept waking up every half-hour or so, each time because the pillow had a new wet spot on it. The cotton ball in my ear had become saturated and fluid had overflowed onto the pillow. The dampness against my cheek roused me. In the dark, I groggily removed the soggy cotton ball, threw it on a mat beside my bed, and inserted a dry one.

In the morning, there were 13 discarded cotton balls on the mat. I was speaking to my sister on the phone later that morning, and I described this scene to her. She was very emphatic: "You need to call the doctor right away. This is not right. Something is very wrong. It's Friday, and if you don't call him now, it will be Monday before you can reach him."

I refused to call. I told her that I had a post-op check-up scheduled the next week, and the doctor wasn't available on Fridays anyway. He was scheduled to be at the university's health clinic only two hours a week. And I was really tired. She kept pressing, and I kept refusing. She's not a medical doctor.

Over the next several days, 24 hours a day, I continued to have to replace the cotton balls. My ear seemed to have an inexhaustible supply of fluid in it. Finally, after about four days, it seemed as if the eardrum had healed enough that fluid wasn't coming out. I saw the surgeon a couple of days later. I told him about the 13 soggy cotton balls. I told him about the continuous fluid leaking over the weekend.

"Oh, that's ridiculous!" he snapped. "That didn't happen!"

I was stunned into silence. He told me that I was cured. I still felt peculiar and I couldn't hear right, but he was emphatic: I was cured.

A week later I was back in to see him. He examined me and concluded that my ear was again full of fluid. Now he was really, really annoyed with me. "How did this happen?" he asked accusingly. I looked at him blankly.

He decided that he was going to slice my eardrum open — again — but this time he was going to put a drainage tube in my ear, open to the outside. A typical patient for this procedure is a toddler. I was in my thirties. I dreaded this solution. It seemed to me that, after this procedure, I would constantly have fluid dripping out of my ear. He scoffed at this concern.

He scheduled the appointment for mid-May, at the very end of the school year. When the day arrived, he had no problem slicing my eardrum open and suctioning out the fluid. However, he was having a lot of trouble getting the tube to stay in. He stepped away for a few minutes to prepare for another try.

When he returned he stopped short, incredulous. He exclaimed, "There's more fluid in your ear!" I did not understand why this fact should be so astonishing. He looked at me as if to demand an explanation. Then he suddenly got very busy — almost frantic. Plans were quickly created: I would be admitted to the hospital for brain surgery a few days later. I was instructed to watch very carefully for signs of infection until then.

It turned out that cerebrospinal fluid was leaking from my brain into my middle ear. There's usually a bone that forms the roof of the middle ear. Apparently, I'd been born without that bone. There was nothing between my middle ear and the membrane surrounding the brain.

Additionally, there was a small hole in that membrane, above the ear, that must have been new. It's not clear why the hole appeared (although I've always suspected that pinching my nostrils shut and repeatedly blowing hard in a futile attempt to clear my ears did the damage).

It turns out that my sister — with no medical training at the time — had a much more appropriate reaction to my report of the facts than the specialist did. It's not surprising that the doctor didn't figure out what was wrong in December or in January or in February or in March. After all, my situation was very unusual.

What is disturbing is that when his mental model and my facts didn't match — when I told him in April about the thirteen cotton balls — he elected to discard the facts and hang on to his mental model. This way of thinking — that the doctor's *theory* trumps the patient's *reality* — could have killed me.

If he'd succeeded in placing the tube in my ear, he would have forced open a direct and quasi-permanent channel from the outside air to the inside of my brain. I almost certainly would have developed meningitis. In fact, I was fortunate that I didn't die in the month between the first time he sliced open my eardrum and the second time.

Throughout this six-month saga I was working hard on my coursework and at the work-study job required as a condition of the full merit fellowship I had been awarded. In May I earned my master's degree. A day or two after the doctor sliced open my eardrum for the second time, the school conducted a ceremony to celebrate graduation. At that event, I was honored with a variety of awards.

The organizers had neglected to tell me ahead of time that I was expected to give a speech in response to receiving one of the awards. I approached the microphone and gave an extemporaneous speech to fifteen hundred people, graduates and guests alike. I spoke about the fact that we *all* had an opportunity to make a difference. I used as my theme the quotation, "Do what you can, where you are, with what you have."[232]

Photos reveal that I attended this event with a cotton ball in my ear.

Then I checked into the hospital. I was scared. I had been told that, as a result of the brain surgery, I might lose the ability to understand — or to use — language. I called my statistics professor, David W. Miller, to talk through the numbers — the odds that I would be seriously and permanently damaged. The clarity he brought was a great comfort to me.[233]

Dr. Kalmon Post, a terrific neurosurgeon, operated on me and saved my life. This exceptional professional appeared as calm, cheerful, and refreshed after performing eight hours of brain surgery as he did before it began. My situation was unheard of and included several complicating factors. He managed the surgery and follow-up care flawlessly, supported by the very attentive staff at Columbia-Presbyterian Hospital in New York.

At the time, I did not know how easy it is for something to go wrong in the hospital. I did not realize how fortunate I was to recover completely and uneventfully.

I hadn't gotten the urgently needed treatment sooner because the other doctor repeatedly dismissed my reports of my symptoms. In one realm in my life, I was winning awards in a competitive graduate school. In another realm, I was treated as if I could not convey the simplest of facts.

Bad Attitude

Recall from Chapter Two that rates of misdiagnosis range from about 1% to 40%. Sometimes your symptoms aren't what doctors expect. Instead of concluding that something is lacking in their knowledge, sometimes they conclude that you are lying, faking, or have a psychiatric illness.

Psychiatric illnesses are important and should be appropriately treated. But telling you that you are mentally ill when what they mean is, "I haven't figured out what's wrong with you," is enough to *drive* the most stalwart person insane. Your experience of your own body is discounted, denied, and dismissed. It's as if you're being told that everything your five senses tells you is a lie.

Discovery Health Channel hosted a television series called *Mystery Diagnosis*. In one episode, a woman who had severe breathing problems was profiled. One of the more striking moments occurred during a visit to a lung specialist.

The woman was asked to blow hard into a tube attached to a machine that measures the flow of air into and out of the lungs. She did so poorly on the test that the doctor rebuked her for not trying hard enough, did not examine her any further, and referred her for psychiatric counseling for her "bad attitude."

Many, many doctors and doctor visits later, after many months had passed and her condition continued to deteriorate, it occurred to someone to x-ray her lungs. She had a large tumor that filled most of one lung. Of course she did poorly on the breathing test. She had a very, very serious lung disease. A psychiatric referral for her "bad attitude" was not a reasonable treatment for a massive lung tumor.[234]

Following Orders

Dr. Jerome Groopman has written a fine — although disquieting — book about diagnostic errors that doctors make.[235] He opens with the story of a woman named Ann who had been getting sicker and sicker for 15 years, and was now skeletal at 82 pounds.

She got sick after every meal. Her doctor was treating her for "anorexia nervosa with bulimia, a [psychiatric] disorder marked by [intentional] vomiting and an aversion to food."[236] Her body was shutting down. She had very serious disorders in just about every organ system. Death was not far off.

She was under strict orders to eat 3000 calories a day — largely cereals, bread, and pasta — in order to gain weight. Ann insisted that she was eating as ordered to, despite the fact that every meal made her sick and resulted in vomiting and diarrhea.

Her doctors were convinced that she was lying about her food intake — otherwise, how could she keep losing weight? Every report of her deteriorating condition simply reinforced their belief in her intractable psychiatric illness, which had clearly continued to worsen despite fifteen years of psychiatric treatment.

Then Ann consulted yet another doctor. She didn't really expect the outcome to be any different from those she'd gotten as a result of seeing roughly thirty other doctors. This one, though, was different. This one listened very, very carefully to her.

After a handful of tests, he concluded that in fact she had celiac sprue, an allergy to an element in many grains. The grain-intensive, 3,000 calorie-a-day diet that her doctor had prescribed was literally killing her. Each meal caused more damage to her internal organs.

A month after this accurate diagnosis, Ann had gained twelve pounds as a result of eating foods to which she was not allergic, foods her body could process and from which it could extract nutrients.

It will take years for her to recover physically and mentally from the ravages of fifteen years of being treated for a mental illness when her primary problem was an allergic reaction to the food she was faithfully eating in a heart-breaking attempt to follow doctors' orders, despite the fact that her body was screaming at her — three times a day — that these meals were destroying her.[237]

If You Say So

One of the many books describing how doctors treat patients, *Wall of Silence,* provides the story of an eight-year-old girl, Elizabeth, who had had kidney cancer. When she told her parents that her cancer had returned, her doctors refused to examine her. They said that she was only seeking attention.[238]

Her mother, at the doctors' direction, ignored Elizabeth's reports of pain and insisted that she engage in normal activities despite the obvious distress she was in. Over three months, the child lost about a third of her body weight. Her mother called the doctors almost two dozen times. Without ever examining their patient, they continued to tell her mother to ignore Elizabeth's attention-seeking behavior.

When she became almost entirely non-responsive, her doctors sent her to a psychiatric ward. When she had a seizure, they finally ordered an MRI, which showed that the cancer had long since spread to her spine and brain.

Grueling treatment over most of the next year saved her life. However, the delay of many months caused by her doctors' refusal to consider that she might be accurately reporting her symptoms — and that the cancer had returned — left her permanently paralyzed from the waist down.[239]

Restless Legs

RLS (Restless Legs Syndrome) is a physical disorder characterized by extreme discomfort in, and an overwhelming urge to move, one's legs. Mild cases may need no treatment at all. People with severe cases of RLS are often chronically sleep-deprived because the condition worsens at night and often makes it nearly impossible to sleep. Sitting in an airplane, a movie theatre, a restaurant, a meeting, or a car can feel like torture.

People with serious cases often end up managing their affairs in order to avoid being expected to sit still, with notable consequences for their professional and personal lives. The Mayo Clinic notes that RLS can be "incapacitating."[240] Until recently, there were no approved treatments for it. Many doctors had never heard of it.

Some people have RLS all their lives, but many develop it as they age. One such man started to have trouble when he was in his 60's. He would get ready to go to bed, but the moment he lay down, the sensation in his legs became unbearable.

This experience is a hallmark of RLS. He would have to get up and walk around to get any relief. The moment he lay back down, the sensation was once again unbearable. After some weeks of this, at wit's end, he went to the doctor. His doctor could find nothing wrong, and after several visits told the man that he wanted to commit him to a mental institution for 30 days "for observation."

The man was already distraught and not thinking clearly as a result of severe sleep deprivation and the bizarre experience he was having every night. He was so upset at being labeled "crazy" that he went home and killed himself.[241]

Three months later, his widow read an article about RLS and realized that it described her husband's experience perfectly. He had died because his doctor, instead of saying, "I don't know what you have, but we'll keep looking until we figure it out," said, in effect, "I know everything about medical conditions. Since what you have doesn't match my knowledge, the most likely explanation is that you are insane."

What Matters

Even when it isn't fatal to act as if the doctor's perspective is the only legitimate one, such a mindset can cause grievous physical and psychological harm to patients. An article in the *New York Times* describes first-hand the heart-wrenching case of a doctor who herself was prescribed a drug that resulted in debilitating side effects.[242]

She and her colleagues often prescribed a particular drug to treat mental disorders. If anyone brought up the fact that weight gain was a side effect, the doctors all dismissed that point as unimportant. Then she herself was prescribed that drug — something she didn't want her colleagues to know.

"'I gained 45 pounds. And my skin got bad. I used to be thin and attractive. Now look at me!' Tears welled in her eyes." She noted that she was constantly exhausted, a known side effect of the drug. "'Now, I have trouble getting out of bed. . . . I drive home and just want to nap. I used to have a great body and jogged five miles four times a week. But the worst part is, I can't get a date. Doctors don't think that's a big issue, but it is. . . . Colleagues tell me, 'Watch what you're eating, lay off the doughnuts, join a gym. . . . If they only knew.'"[243]

She is not the only person to discover, too late, that her view of the trade-off between risks and benefits is not at all the same as her doctor's. Said another way, the woman in this story felt that her life had been ruined by the treatment she was given.

Two Sizes

Recall that most doctors don't discuss side effects with patients. People may be embarrassed about their weight gain and not connect it to their drugs.

A number of years ago, a doctor changed a prescription I was taking. Right before he did so, it happened that I had bought a new pair of slacks. I left them to be hemmed. After a couple of weeks on the new regimen, I went back to pick up the slacks. They were now two sizes too small.

I never talked to the doctor about it. I didn't make the connection. I was also embarrassed. I hadn't changed my diet or exercise routine — and I was very active — but nothing in my closet fit.

It was only when I talked to an internist at work almost a year later that the light dawned. "Elizabeth!" he said, "You've gained 15 pounds since I last saw you! What's happening?" I told him that I didn't know, and started describing various minor medical events of the preceding year. When I got to the drug change, he immediately said, "Oh! That accounts for it. That's a well-known side effect. Fifteen pounds. Nothing you can do about it."

Then I was angry. My doctor's choice of treatment had led to a change in my body that to me was major and unwelcome. It had an impact on my mood, on my health, and on my wardrobe. Surely the doctor had known about this side effect — but he didn't discuss it with me. Even when I went back periodically for check-ups, he didn't say anything about the obvious weight gain.

I felt violated — someone had done something to the inside of my body without my knowledge or consent. Even if there had been no other treatment choice — a questionable supposition — forewarning me would have made the situation much easier to deal with. Clearly, this side effect and its impact on me were not considered important.

How could I be in charge of managing my own health without knowing the cause of that weight gain? People have to occupy the bodies being treated 24 hours a day, 365 days a year. When they are treated with unthinking disregard of this fact — and the fact that treatments have downsides — it can create a sense of helplessness and hopelessness.

That's not a picture of a health care system that is focused on meeting your needs. That's a picture of a health care system that may create big obstacles for you if you try to take responsibility for your health.

Difficult Patients

Sometimes the lack of regard that many doctors have for how their patients experience their health plays out in more subtle ways. For example, doctors consider some patients "difficult." Does that mean that they have complex cases that require extraordinary skill to address? No, when doctors talk about difficult patients, they usually mean that they don't like the patients' attitudes.

In an article in *Health Affairs*, a doctor describes three difficult patients.[244]

The first patient wanted to self-manage his insulin-dependent diabetes without a lot of testing and follow-up from his doctor. His physical condition was excellent, and the doctor reports that even his blood sugar level was "not too bad for a do-it-yourselfer." He had been taking care of himself with little medical intervention for *fourteen years*, with good results. He wanted to come in once a year for a check-up and prescription refills.

The doctor was incredulous: "What self-respecting physician would relinquish total control of a complex illness to a patient? None that I know." The patient is viewed as "difficult" because he wants to be the one in charge of managing his illness.

The doctor assumes that it is his (the doctor's) ball game and his ball field, so to speak. The doctor, at this point in the story, has known the patient for five minutes. Yet he sees it as *his* prerogative to "relinquish" or not "relinquish . . . control" of this man's illness to the man himself.

The second difficult patient was a member of the "worried well." This elderly woman wanted to get every new test she heard about; she called the doctor day and night with minor concerns that she magnified all out of proportion, and was constantly convinced that she had some unspecified dreaded disease despite the doctor's repeated assurances. Assume that he's completely correct and that she really is fine.

What is she guilty of? Buying into the ideas that:

- Health care is about delivering tests and treatments.
- Any imperfection, no matter how minor, requires medical attention.
- The doctor is the one in charge of her well-being.

She actually represents a logical end-point of many of the unspoken assumptions that the health care system fosters in patients.

The third difficult patient is a man who hurt his neck at work a year earlier. Initially he was optimistic about every treatment prescribed, assuming that he would soon be able to resume his normal life, including his job. But he has been defeated by a year of constant pain and the failure of treatment after treatment to help him. He radiates misery.

The doctor writes, "A patient has to believe in his doctor and vice versa. . . . [The man] has given up on me and himself. Neither of us has any expectation now that I will fix his damaged neck." He is a "difficult patient" because, after twelve months of fruitless treatment, he doesn't "believe in his doctor."

The doctor has come up with labels for his three patients. The man with diabetes is "a know-it-all." The woman who wants every minor ailment addressed is "a hypochondriac." The man whose injury has obliterated his former life is "a pain in the neck."

The doctor is clear about his point of view. It is less evident that he appreciates his patients' perspectives. He is prepared to say even how they should feel: the "know-it-all" should feel *more* worried; the "hypochondriac" should feel *less* worried, and the "pain in the neck" should feel optimistic.

A Family Affair

Sometimes it seems as if individuals and their families are viewed as obstacles in the delivery of care, rather than as critical elements in it. Their participation is presumed to interfere with the work of the professionals, as if that work can be conducted almost without reference to the patients and their lives.

That perspective fits perfectly with the idea that health care is about delivering acute interventions. It doesn't fit very well with the idea that health care is about getting you good results.

Consider the role of family members when individuals are hospitalized. Historically, family members have been viewed with suspicion, and great efforts have been made to limit their involvement. In fact, in an earlier era, even when children were hospitalized for months, parents were permitted to see them for only an hour or two each week.[245]

Even today, visiting hours may be severely limited. A spokesperson for an organization that advocates family involvement notes, "If we could make only one change in health care, it should be to change the notion that families are visitors. Families are allies and partners for safety and quality."[246]

The biggest problem with the patients-and-families-as-obstacles view is that it isn't supported by the facts. Consider the experience of one hospital in which family-friendly policies were about to be put in place. Doctors and nurses resisted. They assumed that no benefit could result. They objected that "family involvement would take up valuable time."[247]

What actually happened? The number of days that patients had to stay in the hospital was cut in half, medical errors dropped by 62%, patient satisfaction increased from 10% to 95%, and nurses enjoy their situation so much that there is actually a waiting list of nurses who want to be hired to work there.[248] In other words, every reported measure of outcomes got better.

That's entirely predictable. When you include in the discussion the people who are directly affected — instead of just unilaterally doing things to them — the results are usually better. That's a lesson businesses have been applying for at least the last 60 years.

While there are, doubtless, individual cases in which unreasonable family members are disruptive, it's not appropriate to use that as an excuse to routinely exclude all families. Of course, family involvement by even very thoughtful family members can also interfere with treatment — if what the professionals are doing does not appear to be in the best interests of the people being treated, and if patients and their families challenge them.

Other hospitals report a similar discrepancy between the suspicions and fears that doctors and staff members had about family involvement and what actually happened when families were allowed a larger role.

For example, one hospital set up a system to allow family members to summon "rapid-response teams" to the patient's bedside if they felt that something was wrong and it wasn't being addressed. What were the professionals' worries about the system before it was implemented? "'We heard people say that this would lead to calls to pick up dirty linens.'"[249]

What actually happened? In every case when family members called for help, the patients were transferred to the ICU (Intensive Care Unit). That is, the patients were in serious trouble and needed immediate attention.[250]

Think about the assumption that people will waste the professionals' time and will focus on minor, frivolous, or irrelevant issues. Does it suggest to you that individuals are viewed as intelligent, capable people interested in getting the best outcomes? Or does it suggest instead that they are viewed as incompetent, self-centered, disruptive bumblers who can't understand the difference between dying and housekeeping?

Dying Wishes

Doctors often simply disregard what individuals have made very clear that they want or don't want near the end of their lives. That disregard is another indicator of the minor role individuals play in health care, in the eyes of the professionals. Even after work is done specifically to get doctors to pay more attention to what people want, they continue to behave in ways inconsistent with individuals' wishes.[251]

"After 25 years of public outcry over the right to die with dignity, doctors are still ignoring patients' last wishes, according to a new study of terminally ill patients."[252] That observation was made years ago. Unfortunately, many people would tell you that it is as current today as it was when it was written.[253]

Blue Eyes, Brown Eyes[254]

The day after Martin Luther King Jr. was shot in April, 1968, Jane Elliott, a third-grade teacher in all-white Riceville, Iowa, decided to teach her students the meaning of discrimination by giving them a two-day personal experience of how it felt to be discriminated against, and how it felt to discriminate.

She divided the class by eye color. The first day, blue-eyed children reigned supreme. She told the class that blue-eyed people are better, cleaner, and smarter. She gave them extra recess and first place in the lunch line. Brown-eyed children were not allowed to play with them during recess.

Every time a blue-eyed child did something smart or otherwise positive, she pointed it out as proof that all blue-eyed people are smarter or better than brown-eyed people. Every time a brown-eyed child did something less than perfectly, she used it as proof that all brown-eyed people are inferior. The second day, she reversed the roles.

The children got the message. What's also very interesting is the impact that the experience had on their work. Academic performance dropped markedly on the day that the children were treated as incompetent and inferior. Academic performance soared on the day that they were treated as if they were intelligent and capable.

Think about the impact on individuals who are routinely being treated by the health care system as if they are ignorant and incompetent even concerning topics on which they are the experts — because the topics are their own symptoms and responses to treatment.

It is reasonable to suppose that being treated that way hampers individuals' ability to behave as competent grown-ups in managing their health and health care — and lessens their desire to do so. Being discounted and marginalized is not good for your health.

CHAPTER NINE

Torture

When you are sick, nearly naked, afraid, and uncertain about what is happening, the heedless behavior of some health care professionals can lead you to feel as if you are being tortured or held hostage. Clear parallels to Stockholm syndrome can be drawn.

Thanksgiving

We were out of town for the holiday. My husband, Stephen, came down with food poisoning, and was in the bathroom all night long, two or three times an hour, with vomiting and diarrhea. Around 5:00 a.m., no let-up in sight, we decided to go to the emergency room.

The doctor examined him and said, "He'll feel much better once we get some fluids and anti-nausea medicine into him." A nurse came in and explained that they could give the anti-nausea medicine either as an intramuscular injection (like a flu shot) or via an intravenous line (IV). They decided to do it via IV. He needed an IV anyway, and the nurse said, "If we put the medicine in the IV, it starts working right away; with an injection, it takes 15 minutes."

Stephen immediately said, "Please give me the intramuscular injection with the anti-nausea medicine. Then please call a phlebotomist or someone else whose job is to stick needles in people's veins all day long. No one else can find my veins."

The nurse laughed, saying in a patronizing way, "Oh, don't you worry. We know what we're doing. We'll have the IV in in no time. You'll see; it will be much faster to put the medicine in your IV. That's what we're going to do."

Stephen replied, "I'm sure you know what you're doing; but the only people who've ever managed to find my veins are phlebotomists. A lot of people have tried; they have never succeeded. Please, get someone who has this as the focus of their job. It's very painful for me to be repeatedly stuck with needles without their ever reaching the vein — I feel like a pin cushion. And by the time you get a phlebotomist here, the intramuscular injection will have worked. Please give me the injection and call a phlebotomist."

"Oh, no, honey, we're going to take care of you. Don't you worry about it. We know what we're doing."

An hour later, here's where things stood:

- They had still not succeeded in getting the IV line in.
- They had not given him the anti-nausea medicine; his vomiting and diarrhea continued.
- Half a dozen more people, none of whom was a phlebotomist, had come in and stuck him with needles several times each, all repeatedly trying to find a vein and all failing, and all remarking in a gee-golly tone how hard it was to find his veins.

Finally — grimacing, writhing, and crying from the hour of constant pain they had inflicted on him — he cried out, "Stop! Stop it! Stop trying! You can't do it!"

The nurse said, in a fake sweet tone, "Now, don't say that. You have to cooperate. Don't you want us to help you?"

It is hard to catalogue the elements of psychological torture in her behavior, but I will try:

Stephen was made to feel invisible in at least two ways. First, he was treated as if he were not even competent to report his own medical history. Stephen had 40 years of experience with his own body to draw on; she had less than a minute. She treated him as if her one minute made her more of an expert about his body than his 40 years did.

Second, the nurse made decisions for him that went against his stated wishes when there was another ready alternative that he emphatically preferred. He repeated his requests several times during the hour. She repeatedly dismissed them.

He was powerless. He was made to feel that facts and logic didn't even enter into the equation. Even when what he said was demonstrated to be true, and he was clearly in a world of hurt, there was no change in the nurse's approach.

It started to feel like he was being subjected to a power play rather than to medical treatment. At that point, miserably sick and in treatment-induced pain without any treatment-induced benefits, he had to have been close to surrendering any sense of dignity or identity that he had started with.

When he made the perfectly rational plea that they cease hurting him, the nurse twisted the situation so that he was supposed to be at fault: "You have to cooperate." He had certainly done so by tolerating being used as a practice pin cushion, in between bouts of vomiting and diarrhea.

Now he was supposed to think that he was the bad guy and they wore the metaphorical white hats. The final insult was her closing line, "Don't you want us to help you?" Of course he wanted them to help him. But this wasn't a situation in which the benefits of treatment outweighed the patient's distress during its delivery. This was a situation in which there would never be any benefits from the approach they were taking, and this fact was abundantly clear.

Expecting him to adopt a mental model in which being physically and emotionally abused equaled being helped was so ugly that it almost made *me* throw up.

I was discounted as well. Shortly after we were put in the exam room, I started to feel very nauseous myself. I realized that there was a strong, awful odor in the room that had nothing to do with Stephen or me. I traced it to a piece of medical equipment and went to find a nurse.

"There's a container in the room we're in that has a really foul substance in it that smells awful — it's making me sick. It looks like vomit or something. It's overpowering. Please, can you do something about it?"

"Oh, that's impossible. He's been throwing up. That's all it is."

"No, that isn't what it is. This is a substance in a container in the room that looks like vomit and smells worse. Please, this is not good to have in the room with him."

"That just can't be. You're just smelling him."

"No, I'm not. Would you please come see?"

After many delays, eventually someone came back into the room — without being focused on sticking Stephen — and immediately realized that the room had been used *the previous day* to pump the contents of someone's stomach out. The stomach pumping device and receptacle had not been cleaned in the many hours since that patient had left.

I was treated with the presumption that I was wrong, ignorant, unable to make simple distinctions, and unable to report simple facts. Being treated that way made me, like Stephen, feel invisible, voiceless, and powerless.

I think we both felt a flash of identification with the soldier Ron Kovic in *Born on the Fourth of July*, a movie which highlighted the appallingly lackadaisical and life-threatening hospital treatment of this Vietnam War veteran. There's a scene in which Kovic, helpless in his hospital bed, just dissolves into tears. It wasn't the underlying medical facts of his case that led to his breakdown. It was the way he was being treated.

Eventually, the hospital staff gave Stephen the intramuscular injection. They never did get an IV line in.

Clean Out

Jamie lay in the hospital, prepped for a procedure. He awaited the arrival of a gastrointestinal specialist. The doctor came striding rapidly into the room. He approached the instrument tray, and asked cheerily, "How did the clean-out process go?"

Jamie was dumbfounded. He was there for an upper endoscopy. There is no clean-out process to perform before upper endoscopies, which involve putting a tube down the individual's throat. The gastrointestinal procedure for which there is a clean-out process is a colonoscopy, which involves the opposite end of the digestive system. Clearly, the doctor was preparing to perform the wrong procedure.

Now what? If Jamie said something that made it clear that the doctor was making a mistake, would that fact rattle him so much that he would be more likely to commit an error — like puncturing Jamie's stomach lining — when he put the tube down Jamie's throat?

If he wasn't even paying enough attention to know what procedure he was supposed to be performing, how carefully would he conduct it? How could Jamie phrase his response so that he didn't get hurt? Or should he just rip the IV line out of his arm and make an escape?

Doctors often feel that they are at the mercy of many other people, including the individuals they treat. A common lament is, "If I tell them something they don't want to hear, they'll just go to another doctor." Yet individuals are also at the mercy of doctors — helpless in their hands, often literally, such as when they are under sedation and being operated on.

These are not parallel difficulties. If an individual goes to another doctor, the first doctor may lose a small amount of revenue. If an individual gets crosswise with a doctor, he has a very real fear that his body — his life — is at risk. Individuals need to have a great deal of help in understanding how to interact with the health care system so that this life-or-death power disparity doesn't impede their quest for improved health.

What happened in this case? Jamie's silence apparently alerted the doctor that something was wrong. He stopped suddenly, saying, "Excuse me. I need to study your chart." He left the room, returning a moment later to apologize. Jamie allowed him to perform the procedure. He got the test results, and never went back to see that doctor again.

Stockholm

How exactly is that experience fundamentally different from being held hostage — and knowing that you have to remain in your captor's good graces because your life may depend on it?

Stockholm syndrome[255] is named for a situation in which hostages in a bank robbery in Stockholm came to identify with their captors — and even to protect and defend them. This surprising turn of events has been used to illuminate the survival strategy of the less powerful party in unequal power relationships. The circumstances that set the stage for Stockholm syndrome are:

- "the constant threat to physical and psychological survival
- a condition of helplessness and hopelessness
- isolation and loss of support systems from the outside world
- a context of trauma and terror that shatters previously held assumptions
- the perception that survival depends on total surrender and compliance"[256]

Do you see any parallels between the situation people face in hospitals and the conditions that foster Stockholm syndrome? Using the story from Chapter One of Bob's week-long hospital stay in which he was nearly killed by an accidental drug overdose, consider these factors one at a time from his mother's perspective:

- "the constant threat to physical and psychological survival"

Yes, Bob's life was in constant danger, and Shannon was facing the devastating possibility that her youngest son might very well die.

- "a condition of helplessness and hopelessness"

Yes, when Bob experienced the near miss with the drugs, his parents had not yet gotten access to the surgeon who would save his life. Each day they watched their baby deteriorate further.

- "isolation and loss of support systems from the outside world"

Yes, in this case the sheer time demands of guarding Bob's life left Shannon with little time to connect with others. Even her two other young children had been sent away to stay with relatives. She could not even go home; it was too long a drive from the hospital.

- "a context of trauma and terror that shatters previously held assumptions"

Yes, and this is so clearly applicable to many people engaging the health care system. There you are, leading your normal life. Out of the blue, a life-threatening health problem suddenly occupies center stage. In this case, Jeff and Shannon's third child looked perfectly normal at birth but had a disorder so extreme as to be unfathomable. Health for most of us is like air: we only notice it when we don't have it.

- "the perception that survival depends on total surrender and compliance"

Yes, in Bob's case, his hold on life seemed so fragile that his parents were scared to deviate at all from the instructions they had been given.

It takes just a few days for Stockholm syndrome to take root.[257] Bob had been in the hospital for nearly a week when the drug error took place. One of the characteristics of Stockholm syndrome is that its victims become profoundly grateful for small kindnesses, treasuring them all out of rational proportion. Here is what Shannon said when I asked her if she had told anyone else in the hospital about the drug error:

"No," she said, "I didn't want to get the nurse into trouble. She had been really kind to me the week I was there."

In retrospect, she wishes she'd said something to the nursing supervisor. It's easy to understand why she's reconsidered. After all, she was trading off "not wanting to get the nurse into trouble," for the possibility that other people would be killed by mistake, because the hospital's procedures readily allowed well-intentioned health care workers to make drug dosing errors.

It appears that her initial decision was the result of being in circumstances that can foster Stockholm syndrome. Only when Shannon's son began leading a normal life — when the crisis was over — could she imagine responding differently.

On a related note, "even the most outspoken and assertive among us may suddenly turn meek when we are sick or vulnerable in a hospital, fearing that our treatment will suffer if we antagonize caregivers."[258] That attitude is not surprising, given that "Many physicians are trained 'to think of [them]selves as little gods' and resist patients who question their authority."[259]

One father, Jon, recounts his experience. He was "fired" by his son's doctor, even though he agreed with and followed the doctor's recommendations for the care of his child, who was very ill with Crohn's disease. This disruption in care placed the child at risk.[260]

Apparently the doctor was incensed that Jon asked questions to try to understand what was going on. Jon notes, "I learned that even if you are deferential and humble, you may still be labeled as 'difficult' and blacklisted from care."[261]

The risks of questioning doctors — being labeled "difficult," being fired, and so forth — are very real today. Those risks create big obstacles for individuals who try to engage in the process of their own care (or in that of family members). A hospital chief executive commented, "It's all too common for patients and family members to remain silent when they suspect something is wrong or improper in their care."[262]

Compare that behavior to a description of survival techniques of individuals with Stockholm syndrome: "The defining characteristic of Stockholm syndrome is the tendency to react to threatening circumstances not with the usual fight-or-flight response, but by 'freezing,' as some animals do by playing dead in order to fool predators. Stockholm syndrome is a position of passivity and acquiescence that works in a similar way as a strategy for survival."[263]

On a similar note, another description of Stockholm syndrome says, "Victims are encouraged to develop psychological characteristics pleasing to captors: submissiveness, passivity, docility, dependency, lack of initiative, inability to act, decide, think, etc."[264]

A health care system that fosters that collection of emotions and behaviors in patients and in their families — intentionally or not — makes it difficult for people to act as successful CEOs of their own health and health care.

Violence

Don Berwick, a doctor in the forefront of efforts to fix health care, reports on an experience in which he wasn't allowed to accompany a friend into a medical treatment room, despite the fact that she was terrified and crying, and begged that he go with her.

The health care professionals in that situation made a choice which caused serious and unnecessary emotional harm to the patient. The position they took was not medically necessary. They could easily have allowed the woman to have the comfort of a familiar face during a very frightening ordeal. But they wouldn't even consider doing so.

Dr. Berwick comments, "I find a lot wrong with that picture. . . . What is wrong is that the system exerted its power over reason, respect, and even logic in order to serve its own needs, not the patient's. What is wrong was the exercise of a form of violence . . . [thereby causing] needless harm."[265]

The health care professionals reportedly took a stance simply because it was convenient for them and ignored the extreme emotional distress it caused the patient. Behavior like that does not improve patients' health and well-being. In fact, such behavior appears to be a form of emotional abuse.

The problem with health care is that it's not about you.

CHAPTER TEN

Gods and Mortals

Patients want doctors to be gods, and doctors want to be gods. For both patients and doctors, the unintended consequences of this power disparity are very destructive. Unintended consequences in health care are common, often creating the very problems they are intended to forestall.

Yellow Pages

Although people are often extremely self-reliant, many people also believe that if something isn't working right, the solution lies in the Yellow Pages, so to speak: find the experts and they'll fix it. That's an understandable view but at times a problematic one where your health is concerned. It tends to put too much weight on the role of the experts and too little weight on your own role.

Restricted Access

Many of us have bought into the idea that health care is mysterious and magical. And access to that magic is limited, although we often pretend it's not. Even if you're lucky enough to have great health insurance and live somewhere where doctors provide appointments promptly, access to health care is still restricted in the sense that it appears to be something that's out of your hands; it's the province of experts.

You can't even find out your own cholesterol level unless your doctor says you can. You have to petition the high priests of health care for just about every test and treatment. And if anyone tries to block your access, you may be outraged. Study after study shows that if you restrict people's access to something — kindergarteners' access to candy, for example — they lust after it a great deal more than do people whose access isn't restricted.[266]

And so at times people clamor for health care interventions without knowing — or even asking — if those will actually help them lead a healthier, happier life. That's an unintended consequence of the fact that health care is portrayed as belonging to the experts.

Absolute Power

We expect infallible experts in health care. We expect gods. And doctors try. They try very hard. For some doctors, every death is a failure, a cosmic slap in the face. So they try harder: maybe this next intervention will work![267]

Attempting to be all-powerful — with the ability to preserve life in even the most hopeless circumstances — leads some doctors into a situation suggested by the famous quotation, "Power tends to corrupt, and absolute power corrupts absolutely."[268]

Social science research concludes that "power leads people to . . . fail to understand other people's feelings and desires. . . . Studies have found that people given power in experiments are more likely to rely on stereotypes when judging others. . . . Predisposed to stereotype, they also judge others' attitudes, interests, and needs less accurately. . . . High-power individuals are more likely to interrupt others, to speak out of turn, and to fail to look at others who are speaking."[269]

That description of people in power dovetails with research that shows that doctors typically interrupt patients and take over the conversation after *eighteen seconds*. That's how long you have to explain what's wrong with you before they redirect the conversation.[270]

For an extraordinary account of the creation of power by doctors in the U.S., there is nothing better than Paul Starr's Pulitzer Prize-winning book, *The Social Transformation of American Medicine: The Rise of a Sovereign Profession and the Making of a Vast Industry.*[271]

Enabling Behavior

If we allow doctors so much power over us, silently begging them to be gods, it's not surprising that they make decisions and take action based on their perspective and priorities rather than on ours.

As an analogy: just as co-dependents enable the behavior of alcoholics, patients may enable the behavior of doctors. Perhaps it's not too much of a stretch to say that some doctors are addicted to delivering an ever-increasing quantity of acute interventions; one might say that interventions are their drug of choice. They may cross an invisible line between beneficial and excessive volume. Many patients go along with that behavior. They put themselves at risk by doing so.

As another analogy, consider the victims of financier Bernie Madoff. They saw $65 billion that they thought was theirs disappear.[272]

They did not ask questions about what he was doing with their money. They assumed that his prestige, secret knowledge, impressive connections, and sterling credentials meant that he would successfully deliver what they wanted, despite the fact that he promised financial gains that defied logic. An article discussing the role of his investors is titled: "Madoff Had Accomplices: His Victims."[273]

Individuals who don't ask questions of their doctors — and who simply assume that they will receive incredible benefits from the doctors' secret knowledge — run a risk that they will face similar severe disappointment. Of course, doctors do at times deliver miracles. But taking that outcome for granted is a high-risk proposition.

Here's what one investor who lost millions with Madoff said: "I remember that it was a myth that he created around him . . . that everything was so special, so unique, that it had to be secret. It was like a mystical mythology that nobody could understand."[274]

Does that sound similar to the stance that some doctors take, that their work is so complicated and magical that asking questions is inappropriate because you couldn't possibly understand? And who are you to question them, anyway?

I recall listening to the comments of an official of the American Medical Association at a national health policy conference one year. Here is what I understood him to be saying: health care is too complicated for anyone but doctors to understand. They should just be left alone to practice it. The only way to improve health care is to pay doctors more than they are paid today, and leave to them all the decisions about what diagnostic procedures and treatments to order.[275] His remarks were entirely consistent with the doctors-as-gods framework.

Of course, doctors are not running financial scams like the long-running Ponzi scheme Madoff perpetrated. But, like him, many of them are attempting to deliver perfect results (at the extreme, no one ever dies) when it is impossible to do so.

This conflict can lead some doctors to a defensive stance. Anyone questioning their authority or decisions is discounted or belittled. They may need to feel all-knowing and all-powerful, in order to continue to attempt to deliver on our expectations that they routinely perform miracles.

Managing Gods

"Managing" and "gods" are not two words that go together very often. One doesn't picture saying to a god, "Okay, explain to me the pros and cons of the different options, and I'll select the one that makes the most sense to me. Then you can go ahead and execute that one."

No one interested in preserving her own neck would dream of having such a conversation with a god. And it can be hard to have that conversation with a doctor today. It will continue to be hard until health care shifts its focus to be about you and the pedestals on which doctors stand are not quite as high.

People report that they use cost and quality data to make health care decisions *less* often today than they did five years ago.[276] One possible explanation is that trying to do so just doesn't seem consistent with the realities of interacting with doctors.

To be clear: it's a good idea to use cost and quality data to inform your health care choices. It's just something of an uphill battle, which is why newspapers, magazines, and websites are full of articles with titles like "Learning to Ask Tough Questions of Your Surgeon,"[277] and "Finding a Way to Ask Doctors Tough Questions."[278]

Unintended Consequences

Unintended consequences of expecting doctors to be gods include creating a power disparity between them and you that can make it harder for you to get what you need.

Much of this book so far has detailed unintended consequences of many diagnostic procedures, treatments, and other health-related activities. For example, ICU Psychosis is induced in many patients — with disastrous long-term consequences — when doctors are simply trying to save their lives.

Sometimes it appears that doctors believe that the only consequences of their actions are the ones they intend. This belief would account for the fact, discussed in Chapter Five, that doctors tend to dismiss patients' reports of side effects.[279] They intend for the treatment to help, and side effects don't fit into that picture. This lack of recognition that there is a gap between their intentions and a messier reality seems to be due primarily to a failure of imagination.

Most of the following examples illustrate a particularly perverse form of unintended consequences: *causing* the very problem that the action is intended to *prevent*.

Test Case

People in the U.S. now get more radiation exposure from medical tests such as CT scans than they get from the environment. Per person, the exposure today is six times what it was in 1980. The World Health Organization has listed x-rays as a cause of cancer.[280]

Of the four million people found in one study to have been exposed to high levels of radiation in one year, "About 400,000 of those patients receive very high doses, more than the maximum annual exposure allowed for nuclear power plant employees or anyone else who works with radioactive material."[281]

Japanese people exposed to radiation from atomic bombs during World War II went on to develop cancer at higher rates than normal.[282] Through medical tests, many Americans today are exposed to as much radiation over time as those Japanese people were.

Expert review of the data suggests that "tens of thousands" of new cancers will arise as a result.[283]

Thus, testing intended to help address serious medical problems may cause them.

Antibiotics

The ready availability of antibiotics may have led to a reduced emphasis on hygiene by doctors and nurses in hospitals: "In the old days . . . nurses and doctors were trained not to touch doorknobs, cabinets, curtains and blood pressure cuffs once they scrubbed and/or gloved. But all of that training really went by the wayside in the early '70s, when the liberal use of antibiotics replaced that attention to rigorous hygiene."[284]

Additionally, when germs are bombarded with antibiotics, the weak strains die off but germs which have some natural resistance to the drugs may survive. The resistant germs multiply and become the dominate strains of the germ. They become "superbugs" which can no longer be controlled by antibiotics and which are more likely to be lethal.[285]

Thus, antibiotics — intended to kill bugs and save lives — may be contributing to deaths in at least two ways. First, health care professionals may be less careful to avoid passing on germs than they were before antibiotics were widely available. Second, the over use of antibiotics makes it easy for hard-to-control bugs to thrive unchecked — and kill people as a result.

Breathe Easy

"The use of antibiotics in the first year of life is associated with an increased risk for asthma at age 7, a new study has found, and the reason may be that antibiotics destroy not only disease-causing microbes, but also those that are helpful to the developing immune system."[286] Thus, a common treatment for respiratory problems may lead to future respiratory problems.

Bones and Teeth

My doctor told me that I should walk more, to help prevent osteoporosis. I complied vigorously, going for frequent, fast-paced, four-mile walks. After a few weeks, I noticed a pain in my foot. "Oh, well," I thought, "it will go away."

Weeks went by, and it seemed to be getting worse, not better. Eventually I went to a foot doctor. He examined me and ordered x-rays. Then he diagnosed a stress fracture, a result of all the walking.

My husband, with his usual keen eye, said, "Okay, let me get this straight. You got a broken bone from walking?"

"Yes."

"Which you were doing to prevent osteoporosis?"

"Yes."

"And the reason osteoporosis is a problem is that it can lead to broken bones?"

"Yes."

"So you got a broken bone by doing something intended to prevent broken bones?"

"Well . . . yes."

"And this was a good idea because . . .?"

I scowled. I was glad that he didn't ask me about the gum surgery I needed, apparently because I had taken too much to heart decades of admonitions to "Brush your teeth!"[287]

Preventive actions may lead to the very problems they are intended to forestall.

Bike Space

One study in the U.K. "suggests wearing a [bicycle] helmet might make a collision [with a car] more likely in the first place."[288] Drivers overtaking bicycles left twice the distance between themselves and bicyclists not wearing helmets as they left between themselves and bicyclists wearing helmets. Thus, safety equipment may lead to more accidents.

(Lest you conclude that it's time to ditch the helmets, please note that many bicycle accidents do not involve cars; the rider loses control of the bicycle due to uneven terrain or some other circumstance and crashes. Speaking from personal experience, bicycle helmets save lives in those situations.)

Avocado

Many people attempting to lose weight are advised to follow a low fat diet. However, it turns out that avoiding fat in meals means that a dramatically smaller amount of important nutrients is absorbed by the body. One study showed that seven to *eighteen* times more nutrients were absorbed when fat like avocado was added to a salad.[289]

"Study researchers say they were not only surprised by how much more absorption occurred with the avocado added to the meal, but they were taken aback at how little the body absorbed when no fats were present."[290] Thus, attempts to be healthier by cutting out fat may impair health by reducing absorption of nutrients.

Cleanliness

Kitchens cleaned regularly with sponges or dishrags — and looking spotless — may harbor dramatically more germs than one that is rarely cleaned and looks it. The reason is that swiping the sponge or dishrag over the countertops spreads around all the bacteria that the sponge or dishrag has picked up. Thus, attempting to keep a kitchen clean may cause illness.[291]

(This research doesn't mean that you shouldn't clean your kitchen; it means that it's necessary to be consistent in disinfecting the sponges or dishrags you use.)

Smoke

One company decided to encourage better health habits on the part of its employees. Management started paying employees a special bonus if they quit smoking. Then they found that some non-smoking employees *started* smoking in order to earn the bonus for quitting.[292] An action intended to improve lung health may, for some people, damage it.

Campaign

"For years, many public health campaigns that aimed at changing habits have been failures. Earlier this decade, two researchers affiliated with Vanderbilt University examined more than 100 studies on the effectiveness of antidrug campaigns and found that, in some cases, viewers' levels of drug abuse actually increased when commercials were shown, perhaps in part because the ads reminded them about that bag of weed in the sock drawer."[293]

"A few years later, another group examined the effectiveness of advertising condom use to prevent AIDS. In some cases, rates of unprotected sex actually went up — which some researchers suspected was because the commercials made people more frisky than cautious."[294]

Thus, educational ads intended to remind people to behave responsibly may result in irresponsible behavior.

Red Lights

To improve safety on the road, many cities have installed cameras at busy intersections to photograph and ultimately fine drivers who run red lights. Study after study repeatedly uncovers the same results: fewer people run red lights, yet more fatalities occur as the drivers who stop at the lights are rear-ended by the people behind them.[295] A set-up intended to save lives instead costs lives.

Lies

Patients lie to doctors. Why? They are intimidated by god-like doctors, want to save face, and try to appease the doctors by appearing to be good patients.[296]

Dr. Gregory House, the curmudgeonly diagnostician in the TV series *House*, is known for his dictum "Everybody lies."[297] On the television show, these lies frequently cause delays in diagnosis and treatment. Patients are often seriously harmed as a result because doctors go down the wrong track in attempting to help them. That happens in real life too.

One study showed huge differences between what patients said they did and what they actually did.   "Researchers looked at how patients used an inhaler equipped with a device that recorded the date and time of each use. . . . Seventy-three percent of patients reported using the inhaler on average three times a day, but only 15% actually were using it that often.   And 14% apparently deliberately emptied their inhalers before their appointments" to make it appear that they had used it far more than they had.[298]

"Some researchers estimate more than half of patients tell their doctors they're taking their medicine exactly as prescribed when they're not. In reality, they don't like the side effects, can't afford the pills or didn't understand the instructions."[299]

Remember the discussion in Chapter Five about the four boxes of possible outcomes when individuals take a drug (or receive other treatment). Doctors may think that they're being more efficient by simply focusing on the "treatment works, no side effects" box.

However, one consequence of that choice may be that individuals experiencing one of the other boxes simply decide not to discuss it with their doctors. Perhaps they're uncomfortable telling doctors that their experience isn't what the doctor led them to expect.

Individuals may put their lives at risk by viewing doctors as gods and trying to garner their favor by lying in order to meet their expectations.

Context

What all of these examples have in common is that actions were taken without considering fully the *context* — meaning the interaction between those actions and other people, the environment, or time. The contexts missed in these cases are:

- CT scans: the body's response to cumulative doses of radiation over time
- antibiotics: the long-term reaction of doctors and nurses reducing their vigilance because infections weren't as scary anymore, and the adaptive behavior of the bugs themselves
- asthma: the elimination of good bugs needed for children's immune systems to develop properly
- bones and teeth: the absence of feedback loops which would help people know how far to take instructions like "Walk more!" and "Brush your teeth!"
- bicycle helmets: the change in drivers' behavior when bicyclists wear helmets

- low fat diets: the behavior of the body in processing nutrients from other foods
- sponges and dishrags: the ability of the cleaning tools themselves to spread germs
- smoking: the reaction of the non-smoking employees
- street drugs and unprotected sex: the audience's focusing on the part of the message that they found appealing, not on the part of the message its creators intended to feature
- red-light camera: the reaction of the driver behind the one at the intersection
- lies: the intimidation patients feel in dealing with doctors-as-gods

In health care, much of the context missed is *you*. Said another way, actions are often taken without considering either how you will react to those actions, or their impact on your overall health and well-being. Doctors sometimes act as if you are simply an inert object whose reaction is limited to the one they intended.

Identifying and addressing unintended consequences in health care requires thinking about any given problem much more comprehensively than is typical. It's necessary to think carefully about the entire *process* of care and how all of its parts relate to each other. The next chapter introduces some basic process management ideas.

CHAPTER ELEVEN

There's Many a Slip 'Twixt the Cup and the Lip

Many unintended consequences and other problems in health care arise because processes are not carefully managed. For example, some problems result when the health care system fails to explicitly identify what can go wrong with each step in a process — and then does not take action to address those issues up front. A crash course in a few aspects of process management can help you get better results from health care.

Lots of Problems

Previous chapters have identified many of the ways in which health care delivery is flawed and reasons why it is so. These include:

- Health outcomes in the U.S. are worse than those in other developed nations, and 12,000 people a week in this country are accidentally killed by health care.
- Up to half of the actions that doctors take to diagnose and treat disease either hurt you or at best don't help you.
- Health care is focused on solving the problems of a prior era, not on helping you be a better CEO of your own health and health care.
- Simple steps that could get you much better results are frequently not even on the radar screen; patients are often a footnote.
- Doctors usually don't tell you that many people aren't helped by a treatment they prescribe, nor do they tell you what problems it's likely to cause you.
- It's often hard to find out what is happening while you are waiting for a diagnosis; and the stress caused by the uncertainty is bad for your health.
- Doctors often don't want you to have access to important information in your own medical records. They prefer to keep it to themselves.
- Patients' accurate reports of facts may be dismissed by doctors who are unable to diagnose them; doctors may also discount or ignore issues important to patients.

- The power disparity between doctors and patients can lead patients to feel as if they are being tortured or held hostage.
- Patients want doctors to be gods and doctors want to be gods. The unintended consequences of this mutual desire can damage your health.

That's a lot of problems. Process management can help.

Process

Even if health care were focused on you, it would take concentrated effort to get the best results. Many, many interrelated steps have to work right in order for you to get good health outcomes. This chapter includes:

- examples that show how breaking an activity down into its various steps can help you see ahead of time what can go wrong
- an example of how a continuing care facility "connects the dots"
- a description, with examples, of how you can use FMEA (Failure Modes and Effects Analysis) to *prevent* problems in the first place
- two additional stories and comments

You Take Action

When you seek health care for even a minor problem — say, your knee hurts — you might experience the following steps:[300]

1. You realize that something is wrong.
2. You conclude that the problem is serious enough that you need medical care.
3. You decide where to get treated, e.g., emergency room or doctor's office.
4. Unless it is an emergency, you contact your doctor's office for an appointment.
5. You make logistical arrangements to keep the appointment (e.g., change your schedule).
6. You may do things to feel better before you see the doctor — e.g., take pain relievers.
7. You go to the doctor's office.
8. A nurse asks questions and takes notes.
9. You are seen by the doctor, who asks questions, makes notes, and gives instructions.
10. After you leave, you may go several places to buy things the doctor told you to get — e.g., a drug store to fill a prescription; a medical supply store to buy a knee brace; and a sporting goods store to get ankle weights for exercises.

11. You change your routine based on the doctor's instructions, e.g., take the medicine and do the exercises.

12. After some time, you realize that you feel better — or that you don't.

If you don't, you start the process all over again.

These twelve actions are all steps in a *process*. They need to happen in sequence. That is, you wouldn't fill the prescription, for instance, before you went to the doctor. You wouldn't arrive at the doctor's office, as another example, before deciding that you have a problem that needs attention.

Notice that most of the steps that require action *that departs from a daily routine* belong to you — deciding to go to the doctor, filling a prescription, making time to do the exercises, and so forth. You're the one who has to make changes, not the doctor. You're the key actor.[301]

Many things can go wrong with most of the steps in the process. In fact, each step has its own unique opportunities for problems. Examples of potential gaps focused just on the patient's side of the equation follow. For the sake of illustration, assume that the individual has a condition that does require treatment and that the treatment prescribed is a valid option with a high success rate.

Before the Visit

First, people may not make good choices about when to seek care, both over using and under using services. As discussed in Chapter Two, over use worsens health outcomes; under use has a similar effect.

Second, actions people take to feel better before they see the doctor may mask symptoms or make a condition worse. For example, analgesics may eliminate fever. The doctor may mistakenly conclude that there is no infection when there is one. Doctors typically don't ask if you have done anything to treat your symptoms prior to the office visit. This gap may lead to errors in diagnosis and treatment.

During the Visit

Third, the patient may not repeat to the doctor all the symptoms she just explained to the nurse, believing that the nurse recorded all the information and that the doctor has read it. This transfer of information has many potential gaps.

Fourth, the conversation between the doctor and the patient provides fertile ground for misunderstanding. For instance, one study involved comparing the answers four doctors got when each asked the same patients about the same set of symptoms.

"The variation in the reports of responses to a simple question like, 'Do you have a cough?' was large." The author suggested that responses to more complex questions would, of course, be even more problematic.[302]

Part of this communication gap may have its origins with the doctor. It is also true that patients may be imprecise in their answers. When my husband was three years old, he complained that his foot hurt. The doctor examined him and found nothing wrong. Three weeks later, he collapsed after jumping on a chair, and it was discovered that he had in fact a broken leg — he had just described it imprecisely to the doctor.

If the doctor and patient don't communicate clearly, then conclusions about what's wrong may be incorrect. Then treatments may not work because they're aimed at the wrong problem. Consequences can be dire: "Miscommunications between patients and health care providers are increasing the chances that people who need medical care will be hurt or killed in the process,"[303] said the organization that accredits health care organizations.

Memory

A fifth gap in the process of health care delivery occurs when doctors rattle off instructions which the patient forgets by the time she walks out the door. One study reported: "If you are a typical patient, you remember less than half of what your doctor tries to explain."[304]

Another concluded: "Five minutes after patients left a doctor's office, they remembered only half of what was told to them; and most of what they did remember was [from] the beginning of the conversation. Yet many doctors give therapy instructions at the end."[305]

Understanding

Sixth, patients may not understand health care information they receive. "National studies have found that 'health literacy' is remarkably low, with more than 90 million Americans unable to adequately understand basic health information."[306]

Another study reported that 41% of the patients "were unable to read directions for taking medication on an empty stomach . . . 26% could not read information about the next medical appointment."[307] If the doctor has given necessary instructions and patients don't understand them, they're unlikely to follow them. Their health may suffer.

Execution

Seventh, patients often don't do what the doctor says. One study reported: "Surveys have found that lack of medication compliance among adults with chronic disease can run as high as 65%."[308]   Another concluded: "Overall, 40 percent of seniors reported not adhering to doctor's orders regarding their medication regimens."[309] Similarly, "Clinical research has recorded adherence rates of 30 to 70 percent."[310]

Chapter Five discussed the fact that drugs are often prescribed for people they don't help or who they actually harm. It's not clear, however, what percentage of the time the people who *don't* take the drugs are the ones who *shouldn't* take the drugs.

Ambiguity

An eighth gap in the health care process occurs when patients do not realize that they have questions until they get home or even until several days have passed. Two examples follow.

I was once given the instruction: "Don't lift anything over five pounds." As days went by, I repeatedly realized that I was uncertain how to comply. When I pulled open a heavy door, I wondered how to tell if I was violating the instructions.

The door certainly weighed more than five pounds, but I was not lifting it, I was just pulling it. Still, the force I had to use was more than it would have taken to lift something that weighed five pounds.

When I pulled a file out of a tightly packed desk drawer, I did not think until later that while the file itself weighed only a few ounces, I had to exert a lot of force to tug it free. Was that the same as lifting something over five pounds?

Was it okay to pick up my big dictionary to check a spelling? I had no idea how heavy it was. (I later found out that it weighed seven pounds.) Was stretching okay? It was not lifting, but it used the same muscles. Thus, what surely seemed like a simple instruction to the doctor was not at all clear to me in everyday life.

A second example of the ambiguity gap concerns instructions for drug dosing. If told to take the medicine an hour before meals, what happens if you have a snack — for example, chips and dip — an hour before dinner? Does the instruction mean to take the drug on an empty stomach? What constitutes an empty stomach?

If you realize belatedly that you have just had a snack without having taken the medicine an hour earlier, now what? Is it better to skip the dose or go ahead and take it on a stomach full of chips and dip? Is the drug just less effective or is it actually dangerous if taken with food?

If the medical advice actually matters, then it is in the details like these that health care either succeeds or fails. If people do not know or cannot get the right answers, they will be acting at cross-purposes to the doctor.

Buy-In

A ninth gap that may occur in the health care process is that patients may understand the instructions but not why they matter. People are given advice constantly, from "Read the instruction manual before turning the equipment on," to "Vacuum the refrigerator coils every six months." Most people appear to ignore most of the advice, and frequently nothing very serious seems to happen as a consequence.

One study showed that 44% of us have ignored a doctor's advice about treatment. Interestingly, 89% said that nothing bad happened as a result. But that means that 11% ended up with a worsening medical problem because they ignored their doctor's advice.[311] And others may have ended up with problems that they just didn't know about yet.

It's apparent that without a clear understanding of their medical condition and its consequences, many people do not take the treatment plan seriously.

Simple Steps

These gaps do not exhaust the list. They are *examples* of the types of problems that commonly occur in even the simplest of health care processes. Any *one* gap can derail health care. For instance, if you forget what your doctor tells you before you even get home, you can't possibly follow her instructions.

In a process with many steps, any one of which can cause the process to fail, the chances of getting good outcomes — in this case, optimal health — are slim unless care is taken to make sure that every step works as intended.

Test Steps

More complex health care situations have a correspondingly greater potential for something to go wrong. For example, add to the equation a single diagnostic test. Additional steps might include:

1. The doctor figures out the right test to order.
2. The doctor's office staff gets insurance authorization, if necessary.
3. The doctor talks with the individual to explain the test, to gain agreement to do it, and to instruct her to schedule it.
4. The individual schedules the test and arranges to be available at the appointed time.
5. The individual follows pre-test instructions. (E.g., "Don't eat for six hours before this test.")
6. The individual shows up at the test site as scheduled.
7. The test site collects the data correctly. (E.g., the test site employee samples the appropriate cells or collects enough blood to be tested and preserves it properly.)

8. The test site performs the analysis correctly. (E.g., the lab technician does the lab work correctly or the radiologist reads the mammogram accurately.)

9. The test site records the results correctly under the right patient's name.

10. The test site reports the results effectively to the physician.

11. The doctor receives and reads the report.

12. The doctor interprets the results appropriately.

13. The doctor notifies the individual of the results.

14. The doctor recommends further testing or treatment if the test results warrant it.

Processes often involve *hand-offs* from one person to another. Notice above that several different people/organizations — the doctor, the doctor's staff, various people at the test site, and the patient — have to take action.

It's easy to see that a misstep at any point can derail the entire process. For example, suppose that the doctor accidentally checks the wrong box on the form to order a blood test. The individual can show up for the test. The lab can perform it and report on it. When the patient is told "Your blood test was normal," she believes that everything is fine. In fact, she could have a serious problem that the correct test would have revealed.

One study concluded that there is "one testing mistake per 30 office visits."[312]

Assume that a process has twelve steps. Assume that each is performed correctly 95% of the time. The probability that the entire process is completed correctly is 54%.[313] That is, something is likely to go wrong nearly half the time. And most real-life health care processes contain far more than 12 steps. Remember that the examples above describe a simple office visit and a single diagnostic test.

Toenails

Some organizations are extraordinarily good at identifying and managing all the steps that need to be taken in order to achieve the best possible health outcomes. Here is one example; it is a small example, chosen to illustrate how attention to even tiny details can make a huge difference:

Medford Leas is a "continuing care" retirement community in New Jersey. Residents may live in houses, in apartments, in assisted living, or in a wing set up like a nursing home. The level of care they get is matched to their needs. People typically start out living independently. As their needs change, they can move to a different housing arrangement that provides for more care.[314]

The retirement community oversees medical care for all residents, regardless of what type of housing they live in. And a podiatrist cuts the toenails of many of the residents. What?

That sounds more like a beauty parlor option than a core medical service. But here's how the medical office connects the dots:

1. The biggest predictor of death and disability in their facility is lack of mobility. That is, an elderly person who can't walk around is likely to die sooner than other similar people who can.
2. What often leads to immobility, particularly in people with diabetes, is a small cut or sore on a foot that then becomes infected.
3. One cause of small cuts or sores or blisters on people's feet is toenails that haven't been properly trimmed.
4. Many of the elderly don't have the flexibility or eyesight to manage trimming their own toenails.
5. Therefore, to promote mobility, a doctor trims residents' toenails regularly. Doing so also allows him to check for other foot problems — blisters, for example — that might worsen and lead to immobility.

The facility works very hard to help residents live independently as long as possible. Medford Leas has done a lot of work to *connect the dots* — to understand what outcome is desired (long, healthy life) and then work backwards to figure out all of the steps needed to make that outcome more likely. Connecting the dots does not happen by accident.

FMEA

Failure Modes and Effects Analysis is one of the most useful tools that process improvement wizards have in their tool kits. If you like to feel in control, you may find it eye-opening and life-enhancing. (If you prefer to let the chips fall where they may, you might want to skip this section.)

FMEA has six parts:

1. Identify all the steps in a process (in as much detail as you can stand).
2. Identify what can go wrong with those steps.
3. For each thing that can go wrong, identify:
   a. how serious it is
   b. how likely it is to happen
   c. how likely it is that this problem will cause damage before you realize what is happening
4. Using a simple formula, rank all the things that can go wrong based on how important it is to prevent them. For instance, something that could result in death, that is highly likely to happen, and that wouldn't be noticed until it is too

late would rank high on the list. Something that would result in a minor inconvenience, that is not very likely to occur, and that can be seen coming a mile away would rank very low.

5. Create plans to address the most troublesome risks and implement them.
6. After plans have been in place for a while, reassess the risks. If some items still score high, or new problems have surfaced, repeat the process.

Getting Dressed

Here is a simple example. This one takes a break from health care; it focuses on what people who work in an office do to select clothing in the morning. Assume that the office requires attire that typically includes a jacket or blazer. What can go wrong? While an FMEA would typically include a lengthy list of problems, just three are listed here as examples:

- The skirt/pants or jacket are too wrinkled to wear.
- There's a button missing, a loose fastener, a hem undone, or some other defect.
- They wore their sharpest outfit two days ago, but have a very important meeting today.

How serious, likely, and hard to see coming is each of these? Assume a scale of 1-10 with 10 being very serious, very likely to occur, and very likely to catch you by surprise, blind-siding you. Assign each item on your list three numbers — one for each of these three characteristics — based on your own judgment. There are no right or wrong answers here.

The numbers 1-10 can be used as often as needed. (That is, it's not necessary to rank the items in comparison to each other at this point.) For each item, the three numbers you've assigned are multiplied together to yield a measure of risk.

Figure 2 shows a spreadsheet listing the three examples of potential problems for the sake of illustration.

If you prepare such a chart in a spreadsheet program, you can easily sort the table by how high the numbers in the right-hand column are. The highest number is listed first. Figure 3 shows the results.

Note that the risk numbers in the right-hand column don't mean anything by themselves. What counts here is the *relative* risk. The items with higher scores create more of a problem in getting the task accomplished successfully than do the items with lower scores. The differences between the multiplied scores make it possible to prioritize and to focus on fixing the most important problems first. Some of the items that rank lower might never seem worth fixing.

Getting Dressed
Failure Modes List

Failure	Severity	Likelihood	Surprise	Risk
Wrinkles	2	10	6	120
Sharpest Outfit Already Worn	7	8	8	448
Defect	6	5	7	210

Figure 2

Getting Dressed
Failure Modes Sorted by Impact

Failure	Severity	Likelihood	Surprise	Risk
Sharpest Outfit Already Worn	7	8	8	448
Defect	6	5	7	210
Wrinkles	2	10	6	120

Figure 3

What does this spreadsheet tell us? The most serious problem for these individuals is that their sharpest outfit, perfect for an important meeting, has already been worn this week. It's a big problem (from their perspective) when it happens — it happens a lot and always seems to catch them by surprise.

Notice that "wrinkles" aren't very serious because they can be fixed in a few minutes. Okay, now what?

Now the individuals think through action plans to address the highest-scoring problems. To address the "sharpest outfit already worn" problem, one solution might be: every Friday they will print out their calendar for the coming week. Sunday night they'll look at it and look at what's in their closet. They'll decide what they're going to wear each day, starting with the day having the events for which they most want to look sharp. They'll write their clothing plan on the calendar and post it inside their closet door.

And so forth. Failure Modes and Effects Analysis is an orderly way to prevent process failures from causing big problems.

Taking a Prescription

If you apply the same thinking to health care — whether you actually draw up detailed spreadsheets or not — you can prevent a lot of problems. For example, here are some things that can go wrong with a prescription for a drug you get in the drug store:

- You're given the wrong drug.
- You're told the wrong dose.
- You misinterpret the instructions for how often and how much to take.
- You forget to take it.
- You have a bad reaction to it.
- It interacts badly with something else you're taking.
- It doesn't work for you.

Figure 4 shows how these problems might appear on a spreadsheet.

Sorted from highest risk to lowest risk, the spreadsheet in Figure 5 shows the results. What are some possible solutions to the biggest problems identified in Figure 5?

- You may misinterpret the instructions:
  - Take notes about any drug prescription the doctor gives you.
  - Ask questions about the dosing instructions and write down the answers. For example:
    - Does that mean that I take one pill four times a day?
    - What does four times a day mean? Does that mean breakfast, lunch, dinner, and bedtime?

Taking a Prescription
Failure Modes List

Failure	Severity	Likelihood	Surprise	Risk
Wrong Drug	10	3	10	300
Wrong Dose	7	3	10	210
Misinterpret	7	6	10	420
Forget	10	5	7	350
Bad Reaction	10	3	10	300
Bad Interaction	10	3	10	300
Doesn't Work	10	6	7	420

Figure 4

Taking a Prescription
Failure Modes Sorted by Risk

Failure	Severity	Likelihood	Surprise	Risk
Misinterpret	7	6	10	420
Doesn't Work	10	6	7	420
Forget	10	5	7	350
Wrong Drug	10	3	10	300
Bad Reaction	10	3	10	300
Bad Interaction	10	3	10	300
Wrong Dose	7	3	10	210

Figure 5

- Am I supposed to take this pill with food or on an empty stomach?
- How long do I keep taking this medicine?
- The drug may not work for you:
  - Ask the doctor how and when you will be able to tell if the drug is working for you.
  - Ask what to do if it is not working.
  - Again, write down the answers.
- You may forget to take the drug:
  - Get a pill container with four little cells for each day (morning, noon, evening, bedtime) and put the correct number of pills in the cells.
  - Put the container where you can't miss seeing it.
  - If you won't be home to see the container, consider getting a small portable pill bottle for your pocket or purse with an alarm that beeps when it is time to take the pill.

FMEA can be helpful in getting better results from a wide variety of processes.

Made in Japan

When I was nine years old, I saved up the quarters from my allowance for months, in anticipation of the annual elementary school fair. It was a highlight of the school year. You could play carnival games of skill and win small prizes. You could buy inexpensive toys. You could buy cotton candy and popcorn.

I left the house with my pockets weighed down with quarters. I won lots of little prizes and bought other toys as well. When I arrived home, thrilled with my loot, my older siblings were exasperated. They looked at my collection of goodies and pointed out that they were all marked "Made in Japan." They said, "This is junk. It will fall apart in a few days." They were right.

Fast forward a few decades. Most of the cars, televisions, stereo equipment, etc., that my husband and I have bought were made in Japan. They are highly reliable and seem to last forever. How did "Made in Japan" go from indicating junk to indicating quality? Process management.

After World War II, an American expert in process management named W. Edwards Deming ended up in Japan to do some work for the Allied forces. While he was there, he was invited to talk with Japanese scientists and engineers.[315] He spoke about how to ensure that actions that are performed repeatedly — like making a car — consistently yield excellent results.

The Japanese scientists and engineers latched onto the insight he provided and started applying it in industry. Deming spent much of the rest of his working life providing further guidance to the Japanese. Today a great deal of the credit for Japan's commercial success is laid at Deming's feet.[316]

Process management is a quietly powerful way to make things work better. It can work even in health care, where every patient is unique. FMEA is just one approach to improving processes; the field of process management includes many others.

The Tortoise and the Hare

Process management has some characteristics in common with the turtle (tortoise) in the fable "The Tortoise and the Hare." In the fable the rabbit (hare) makes fun of the turtle's speed, and in response the turtle challenges him to a race. That proposal seems ridiculous. Everyone knows that rabbits are faster than turtles.[317]

If you've ever heard the story, you remember the ending: the rabbit shows off, racing away at high speed. Then he decides that he's so far ahead that he need not hurry. To show his contempt for the turtle,[318] he stops to take a nap. By the time he wakes up, the turtle has crossed the finish line. The moral of the fable is "Slow but steady wins the race."

Similarly, process management is not glitzy. It doesn't get sound bites on the evening news. It doesn't dazzle with its heroics. It just gets the job done. In health care, having the basics done right — getting the right dose of the right drug, for instance — isn't glitzy or dazzling. It may mean the difference between living and dying — but it's not glamorous.[319]

Process Points

A key message of process management is that getting great results is generally not based on having star players who execute dramatic saves. It's based more on being crystal clear about what needs to happen in each step in a process, and designing the work to eliminate chances to do it wrong or to overlook something critical.

Another key message is that when something does go wrong, attacking the individual who made the mistake is unlikely to help. Problems in health care or any other process are not usually the fault of "bad apples." They are usually the fault of bad processes.

Focusing on process management to make things work better is sometimes called "continuous improvement." Dr. Don Berwick, ahead of the curve, noted in 1989: "Usually the failure of a process lies not in the work ethic of the workers, but in poor job design, failure of leadership or unclear purpose. . . . American medicine needs to abandon the Theory of Bad Apples and embrace the Theory of Continuous Improvement."[320]

A consistent theme running through the discussion of process management is that it's important to be clear about the *purpose* of the process — what outcomes you want to get — and then to think through carefully all the little steps along the way that need to be managed to increase the odds of achieving those outcomes. Leaving anything to chance is less likely to yield good results.

CHAPTER TWELVE

Purpose

Most process improvement efforts fail because people forget to ask the most critical questions before they wade in and start trying to fix things. Simple game-changing questions provide a new perspective about the purpose of health care.

Low Down

In August, three years after Bob had the successful heart surgery described in Chapter One, his mother was troubled by health problems of her own.

Shannon's primary care doctor was sure that her symptoms meant that she had MS (multiple sclerosis). It took until January, though, to complete all the testing the insurance company insisted on to confirm that diagnosis before they'd pay for treatment. Shannon continued to get worse over those five months.

In early April, two or three months into a treatment regimen, Shannon felt worse than ever. Each day she sank deeper into exhaustion. In a routine check-up, the neurologist ran blood tests to rule out any unknown problems.

Later that month Shannon was slated to lead a team of friends in a three-mile MS walk-a-thon. The day of the event she dragged herself out of bed and put on a smiling face to greet her team. They all chose to walk at a casual stroll, worried about Shannon's energy level. Even so, she and her walking partner fell further and further behind.

Her teammates assumed simply that the two were so engrossed in their conversation that they forgot to concentrate on walking. It turned out that Shannon was struggling simply to keep putting one foot in front of the other and keep moving.

Having assumed that the gruelingly overwhelming exhaustion would be a feature of her life from now on, and shifting back and forth between despair and acceptance, at the end of May she went to see the neurologist for another regularly scheduled checkup.

The next day she got a call from the doctor's office telling her that she had to come back in right away. Shannon was frightened by the call — she had just been there the previous day. And she knew that her doctor was booked four weeks in advance. What was going on?

When she arrived, the doctor explained that her blood test results from early April showed a condition called pancytopenia, which means that the blood count for all three parts of her blood — red blood cells, white blood cells, and platelets — was dangerously low.

It had constituted a medical emergency. But nothing had been done about it. No one had told Shannon the test results. No one had prescribed any treatment.

The previous day, six weeks after the earlier tests, the doctor's staff had drawn blood as usual. The results of these tests showed an even further dramatic drop in her blood count. When her doctor saw the results and realized that Shannon had clearly been living with this worsening condition for months, she was very upset.

She wanted to hospitalize Shannon right away and give her blood transfusions — her blood count was so low, it could have been life-threatening.

Glad to have an explanation for her grinding fatigue, Shannon was nevertheless frantic. Who would take care of her children with her husband away on a business trip? She did not want to go into the hospital and she was worried about the safety of blood transfusions.

After much discussion, the doctor agreed instead to give her B-12 shots and to monitor her very closely. She was cautioned to avoid all people and situations that might expose her to illness; her immune system could not fight back.

Her doctor also had Shannon temporarily stop taking one of the main MS drugs that had been prescribed for her — the dangerous drop in her blood count was a direct side effect of the drug.

Shannon had two doctors, her primary care doctor and the neurologist specializing in MS. The neurologist had ordered the original test, and the results were sent to both doctors. The primary care doctor believed that the neurologist would make treatment decisions based on Shannon's MS drug regimen.

The neurologist was so busy that the lead time to get an appointment with her was very long, and the primary care doctor was part of the same medical group. Thus, the neurologist expected Shannon's primary care doctor to treat her.

Shannon had endured worsening extreme exhaustion, emotional torment, and potentially life-threatening changes in her blood for much longer than she should have had to, simply because her doctors did not notify her of critical test results the first time. Clearly, their *process* for reporting test results was broken.

Two Really Big Questions

To fix a broken process, it is critical to be very clear about the *purpose* of the process. You can discover the purpose by asking two critical questions:

- Who is intended to benefit from this process?
- What do they want from this process?

Test Results

To illustrate why it's critical to be clear about *purpose*, consider the process of reporting test results to individuals. Delays and failures in this process were highlighted in Chapter Six and in Chapter Seven and in Shannon's story above.

Doctors say that reporting normal test results to individuals takes up too much of their time. However, they do want to tell people personally about abnormal results.[321] Individuals say that they want to receive *all* of their test results. They care most about receiving as quickly as possible any abnormal results, so that they can start dealing with the problem.[322]

Suppose that *doctors* are viewed as the primary beneficiaries or customers of the process. Then the purpose of any proposed fix might be "to save doctors time by eliminating the need to talk with individuals when no further medical action is required."

Suppose, on the other hand, that *individuals* are viewed as the primary customers of the process that notifies them of their test results. Then the purpose of any proposed fix might be "to minimize stress and reduce the failure to treat serious conditions caused by delays or failures in notifying people of their test results."

If the *doctor* is considered the primary customer, then the solution might be a system with two features: first, it reports normal results to patients without the doctor's involvement and without any great urgency — via mail, perhaps. Second, it traps abnormal results and sends them to the doctor's desk. There they might sit and wait for days or weeks — or longer — until he has a chance to call or see the patient.

If *individuals* are identified as the primary customer, then the solution might be a system that reports *all* test results to patients the same day they are available, perhaps either automatically via electronic notification or by phone calls from one of the doctor's staff.

If staff members call people with seriously abnormal results, they could immediately schedule them to come in to meet with the doctor. If the notification is electronic, alerts could be built in so that staff members know to call patients with seriously abnormal results if they don't call in promptly to schedule an appointment.[323]

The two solutions are very different. The differences arise from asking who is intended to benefit and what they want, questions that foster clarity about the *purpose* of the process.

Different Opinions

What is the *purpose* of the health care system? You might be surprised to hear that there isn't a standard, agreed-upon answer to this question.

If you ask a doctor, you might hear: "To diagnose and treat disease."[324] Advocates for the uninsured might say: "To provide access to health care for everyone." Other people will reply: "To give each person the chance to pursue any and all treatments that might help them improve health or stave off death."

Public policy experts typically say: "To improve population health." This means figuring out how to spend the available money to get the best health outcomes for the greatest number of people for the longest period of time. For instance, investing in cleaning up the water supply and creating better sewage treatment systems was a brilliant move a hundred years ago, and continues to be one of the best ways to improve and maintain population health.

Acute Interventions

Having read up to this point in this book, you might conclude that regardless of what anyone says, the evidence suggests that the actual purpose of the health care system today is "to deliver acute interventions." The health care system certainly does that. For example, each year there are:

- 119,000,000 trips to emergency rooms
- 102,000,000 hospital outpatient visits
- 37,000,000 hospital admissions[325]

What happens if you back up a step to ask who the primary beneficiaries (or customers) of health care are? It might be reasonable to conclude that the primary customers of health care are "the people who need/receive care."[326]

What do they want from health care? As suggested in Chapter Three, most people don't want to be patients; they find having an illness or injury — and dealing with the health care system — to be huge and unwelcome disruptions.

As a result, what they want from health care is "to get back to living their normal lives." Putting together those two answers, one could conclude that health care's purpose should be *to enable people to lead the lives they want.*

Of course, you need other things besides health care to enable you to lead the life you want. And there are some very real limits to what health care can accomplish. However, if you ask yourself what role you want health care to play in your life, you are likely to conclude that "to deliver acute interventions" is not good enough.

The emphasis on acute interventions leads doctors to narrow their vision, and to focus on treating numbers (cholesterol levels or blood pressure) rather than to focus on your ability to continue to live in your own house, go to work, drive your car, take care of your children, plant flowers, go on outings with your family, ride your motorcycle, play the piano, travel, manage your finances — or whatever else it is that you want to do.

Sometimes, given the choice, you might elect not to treat a condition, or to treat it less invasively (e.g., exercise instead of surgery), if you knew ahead of time how much the proposed treatment would interfere with your ability to lead the life you want.

An Ounce of Prevention

A front page article in the *New York Times* was headlined "Cancer Group Has Concerns on Screenings." The subtitle read: "Analysis Finds Benefit to Be Overstated." The article leads off: "The American Cancer Society, which has long been a staunch defender of most cancer screenings, is now saying that the benefits of detecting many cancers, especially breast and prostate, have been overstated."[327] The article reports on new research discussed in the *Journal of the American Medical Association*.[328]

Other reports make similar points. PSA (Prostate Specific Antigen) screening tests can show whether PSA levels are high or are increasing rapidly. These results are markers for prostate cancer. The test is considered standard in the United States for men over the age of 40 or 50.[329] However, the screening test "saves few lives and leads to risky and unnecessary treatments for large numbers of men, two large studies have found."[330]

Prostate cancer progresses very slowly, and many men will have long since died of something else before prostate cancer would kill them. It's as if 50 men were told: "You may become impotent and/or incontinent, or your bowel movements may be painful or you may have chronic diarrhea, so that ten years from now, one of you will be alive who otherwise would have died of prostate cancer."[331]

Or, as the chief medical officer of the American Cancer Society said, "The test is about 50 times more likely to ruin your life than it is to save your life."[332] If the purpose of health care is *to deliver acute interventions*, then of course it makes sense to get tested and treated.

However, if the purpose of health care is *to enable people to lead the lives they want*, there's a big question about whether men, understanding the above statistics, would decide to go ahead even with screening, much less with treatment.

Statins

On a similar note, a large number of people who have high cholesterol, but haven't had heart attacks or heart disease, would have to take statins (a drug for reducing cholesterol) for one person to benefit.

One doctor translated the research results as follows: "What if you put 250 people in a room and told them they would each pay $1,000 a year for a drug they would have to take every day, that many would get diarrhea and muscle pain, and that 249 would have no benefit? . . . How many would take that?"[333]

Again, if the purpose of health care is *to deliver acute interventions*, then this treatment makes sense. If the purpose of health care is *to enable people to lead the lives they want*, then people might have a lot of questions about proceeding.

These examples of testing and drugs that may not serve people well are just that — examples. It's entirely possible that further research may show more health benefits for these particular tests and treatments than current science has identified.

The point here isn't these particular examples. It's the idea that it's important to be clear about your *purpose* in pursuing care, and understand whether the available facts about the test or treatment suggest that it is more likely to *help* you or to *hinder* you in achieving your purpose.

Change Process

If the purpose of health care were *to enable people to lead the lives they want* — if health care were to revolve around you — how would efforts to fix health care change?

1. Efforts would start by identifying the steps or phases of health care as they look from the individual's perspective.
2. For each step, the gaps or shortcomings that interfere with people's ability to lead the lives they want would be identified.
3. Issues targeted for improvement would be those that create the biggest obstacles for people in leading their lives.

Fourteen Steps

Here are fourteen steps or phases of health care that individuals might face over time. For the sake of illustration, these assume that eventually a serious illness will develop.

1. Wellness
2. Risk Assessment
   - Given personal and family medical history, are you at greater than average risk for heart disease? For diabetes? For other chronic conditions?
3. Prevention
   - Given the risks identified, are there changes in your life that would be good to make to reduce the likelihood that those risks will turn into problems that prevent you from leading the life you want? These changes might be related to diet, exercise, and/or other daily activities.

4. Early intervention
   - Given the risks identified, would it increase the odds that you can lead the life you want, for as long as possible, if you started treatment to improve health indicators such as blood pressure? Great care is needed to weigh the very real risks of such treatment against the potential benefits.
5. Triggers
   - What symptoms are serious enough that they mean you need to get expert help from the health care system?
6. Triage
   - How do you tell how fast you need to get help? Is it okay to make an appointment two weeks from now after you get back from vacation, or should you go to the emergency room today?
7. Diagnosis
   - What is wrong with you? What's the underlying cause?
8. Interpretation of the meaning and impact of the diagnosis
   - How do you deal with the mental and emotional shock that this abrupt change in your circumstances creates?
   - Does this diagnosis mean that you'll miss an important business meeting you've been working on for six months? Have to skip your best friend's wedding? Never play the piano again? Die before your children are out of high school? Result in other impacts that have great significance to you?
   - How do you modify your life to accommodate this change while still preserving as much as possible your ability to lead the life you want?
   - In other words, how do you wrap your mind and heart and soul around this diagnosis and figure out how to live with it?
9. Selection of treatment
   - What are the reputable treatment options? What are their pros and cons in terms of how they will improve or interfere with your ability to lead the life you want, both now and down the road?
   - What's the best treatment choice based on *your* priorities/values?
10. Preparation for the treatment
    - E.g., if you are having surgery, what do you have to do ahead of time? Do you need to stop taking some medicines? Make changes at home to be ready to cope with limitations as you recuperate?
11. Delivery of treatment
    - Either the care provider takes action such as performing surgery, or you do something yourself such as injecting insulin daily.

12. Post-treatment management
    - E.g., if you've had surgery, what do you need to do to increase the odds that you will heal properly?
    - Now that the realities of the physical change are sinking in, what other logistical problems need attention? E.g., if you are temporarily in a wheelchair and can't reach the kitchen cabinets, how do you manage meals?
    - What emotional impact is this change having on you, and how do you accept and move through that? For example, for many people it feels as if the earth has moved if they suddenly end up in the hospital with a serious problem. They had not given much thought to their health, but on a subconscious level assumed that they were invincible. Suddenly they can no longer trust that their bodies will keep on performing as usual. It can be an enormously unsettling experience.
    - What are the spiritual implications of this change in health and of the treatment? Many people find that a serious illness leads them to rethink their life focus and priorities.
13. Feedback loop
    - Did the treatment work? Did it solve the problem it was intended to solve, increasing your ability to lead the life you want?
    - Did it cause other problems? If so, what has to be done to address those?
14. Integration of episode of care into life
    - Does this condition — and its treatment — change the answers to the questions in any of the earlier steps? E.g., does it change the triggers which indicate that you need medical care, or how fast you need attention if something goes wrong?

The above list might strike some people as unusual; it has so much in it about individuals and their lives. Yes, it does. That makes sense if the purpose of health care is *to enable people to lead the lives they want.*

Consider what Dr. Don Berwick, a proponent of individual-centric health care, had to say: "I have come to believe that we — patients, families, clinicians, and the health care system as a whole — would all be far better off if we professionals recalibrated our work such that we behaved with patients and families not as hosts in the care system, but as guests in their lives."[334]

Below are examples of how clarifying the purpose of health care would lead to shifting the spotlight to steps (or aspects of steps) that are neglected today. The examples involve the following steps:

- step #7 — Diagnosis
- step # 8 — Meaning and Impact
- step #13 — Feedback Loop

Diagnosis

As discussed in Chapter Two, studies of autopsy results suggest that misdiagnosis is a factor in deaths perhaps 20% of the time. Many of those who die in these cases would probably live if they were treated for the condition they actually have.[335] (Deaths due to misdiagnosis are not counted in the deaths that result from health care, as calculated in Chapter One.)

Clearly, people cannot lead the lives they want if they are dead. They also cannot lead the lives they want if they are in a downward spiral of misery because they are enduring side effects and complications of treatment after treatment — ordered by their doctors as they continue to deteriorate over time — with little chance that any of the actions will actually help.

Further, anecdotal evidence suggests that many people who eventually get an accurate diagnosis may spend months or years in the health care system before they reach that point.

Right now, the topic of delayed and incorrect diagnoses is scarcely on the radar screen.[336]

If the purpose of health care were *to enable people to lead the lives they want,* then one focus of process improvement might be to improve dramatically the speed and accuracy of diagnosis. It is true that it can be almost impossible to reach a diagnosis in some cases.[337] That said, it is likely that misdiagnoses — and lengthy delays in arriving at accurate diagnoses — would be much less common if serious efforts were made to prevent them.

One task would involve figuring out how long it typically takes to get from the patient's first report of symptoms to an accurate diagnosis, for a handful of selected medical conditions for which diagnosis is often problematic. Another task would involve analyzing what happened in that time — what false starts or missteps occurred that resulted in delays in getting accurate diagnoses, and why they occurred. Then solutions could be created to address those problems.

Meaning and Impact

Shannon's experience after being diagnosed with multiple sclerosis provides an example of issues with meaning and impact that provide fertile ground for process improvement.

Shannon works hard to enhance the lives of a wide variety of people. She is Supermom to her three elementary-school-aged children. She is a leader in their schools, her church, and the community. She not only volunteers for many programs, she's usually the one leading the initiatives. Her identity — her self-definition — is all about serving others. That is what her life is about and that is what gives her satisfaction.

Her disease has flared up more often and more severely than is typical. It's hard to know why for certain, because multiple sclerosis is highly variable from one person to the next. That said, it is likely that a factor contributing to the flare-ups is that she is constantly exhausted.

Exhaustion is a characteristic of the disease itself. However, Shannon has a schedule that would exhaust the most robustly healthy person, because she rarely says no to any request for help or to any plea to lead a service project. Other people come first.

When there's a conflict between her identity and the medical advice she is given, it's understandable that she typically comes down on the side of preserving her self-definition. As a result, she simply doesn't get around to all the steps that she needs to take to optimize her health, because they appear to conflict with who she is.

One of the guidelines she was given was: "Take a rest day between days of high activity." She laughed in exasperation as she described her reaction to hearing this advice. "I have three young children. My husband travels on business. How exactly is that supposed to work?"

It is relatively easy for her to take the drugs she is prescribed. Doing so doesn't interfere with other activities very much. It is relatively harder for her to take some of the time that she puts into volunteer activities and use it to rest instead, which would help manage the exhaustion. She gets no satisfaction from resting; she loves the volunteer work she does, and cherishes the time she spends actively engaged with her children.

Because she is still working through "meaning and impact," doing things that are consistent with her self-identity but not with the demands of the disease, no drug can possibly help her very much.

Shannon is not the first person to be given a diagnosis of a serious disease. Clearly, expecting each individual to figure out from scratch how to think about its meaning and impact is a wildly inefficient approach to health care. A question worth asking might be: how have other people with this condition managed the conflict between their self-definition and the demands of the disease?

The absence of guideposts or experienced companions to help lead the way can have only one result: increased stress and long delays in figuring out how to deal with the illness. For instance, at one point Shannon was worried that some of her symptoms might mean that she shouldn't drive. It was an answer she didn't want to hear. As a result, she was afraid to ask the question.

Finally, she hesitantly mentioned it to her doctor, and immediately discovered two things. First, the symptoms she was worried about had no bearing on her fitness to drive. Second, they could be readily addressed through physical therapy. But she had gone through months of anxiety worrying about this situation. That stress clearly was not good for her health.

Doctors, nurses, and others don't usually *anticipate* and address patients' fears. That fact reflects a big gap in health care.

It is not hard to guess what some of the questions are that many people newly diagnosed with a serious disease might have:

- Will I be able to . . .
  - Work?
  - Take care of my children/spouse?
  - Have sex?
  - Walk?
  - Drive?
  - Engage in sports or other activities?
- Will I have normal bowel and bladder function?
- Am I going to have a lot of pain?
- How much will treatment interfere with my life?
- What will happen to my energy level?
- Am I going to be disabled?
- How am I going to pay for it?
- How will this diagnosis change how my family and friends and boss and co-workers treat me? How do I talk with them about it?
- How is having this disease going to change my concept of who I am?
- Am I going to die before I otherwise would have?

Perhaps doctors or nurses could offer a list like the above and say, "Some people diagnosed with this condition have questions about topics such as these. Which ones are you concerned about? What others, not on the list, may I help you with?"

To summarize, process improvement efforts related to "meaning and impact" might focus on:

- developing effective ways to help people articulate what matters to them — what lives they want to lead — and ways to help doctors understand how to acknowledge and incorporate that information into care plans
- making it standard practice to offer individuals insight gleaned from the experience of other patients who have walked a similar path — in an efficient way that addresses their specific concerns
- designing approaches to anticipating and addressing the fears that people have
- creating ways to help people truly understand the trade-offs they are making when they choose certain treatments or behaviors: what impact their choices will have on their ability to lead the lives they want, both now and in the future

In Shannon's case, it is clear that the best thing the health care system could do for her is to help her with the issue of meaning and impact. However, that topic does not even seem to be on her doctors' radar screens. They appear to be focused on choosing between Drug X and Drug Y.

Feedback Loop

A basic tenet of process improvement is that it doesn't work simply to do something and never look at what happens as a result.

In health care, an astonishing percentage of the time, no one checks to see if the actions taken got the intended results. They may verify that, yes, the drug was prescribed or the surgery was performed. These are appropriate feedback loops if the purpose of health care is *to deliver acute interventions*.[338] They are not sufficient if the purpose is *to enable people to lead the lives they want.*

One doctor and researcher, David Eddy, points out how little is known about the outcomes of treatments. An article in *Business Week* titled "Medical Guesswork" chronicles his efforts to illustrate this point.[339]

He would go to annual meetings of different specialists — perhaps orthopedic surgeons or heart doctors. He would ask the doctors there to suppose that a typical patient was given a specific common treatment. Then he would ask them to write down the probability of a particular patient-centric result.

He asked urologists, for instance, what the odds were that a man could urinate normally after surgery to treat an enlarged prostate. "The results were startling. The predictions of success invariably ranged from 0% to 100%, with no clear pattern."[340]

That experience alone is evidence that the health care system behaves as if its purpose is to deliver acute interventions: the process is concluded when the intervention is delivered. What actually happens to patients' ability to lead their lives as a result of the intervention is not typically tracked.

If the purpose of health care were *to enable people to lead the lives they want,* then process improvement efforts might focus on creating a feedback loop and using the information gained to improve care.

Doctors would have to ask up front what the treatment is intended to help the patients do in their lives. Doctors and patients would need to be clear about whether the treatment can, in fact, deliver those benefits. (If a middle-aged woman wanted knee surgery with the hope of becoming a ballerina, the surgeon might want to negotiate a more realistic goal.)

As with goals in business, this approach works best if the goals are agreed to by both parties, are written down, and are SMART:

- **S**pecific
- **M**easurable
- **A**ctionable
- **R**ealistic
- **T**ime-Bound[341]

For example, if a woman is having a knee replaced, one of her SMART goals might be something like: "Three months after surgery, to be able to walk two miles up and down the hills in my neighborhood in 40 minutes or less without any assistive device (such as a cane) and with no more pain than can be managed with one 400-mg dose of ibuprofen."

Once the expectations are agreed upon between the doctor and the patient, the treatment could proceed. After treatment, the agreement would form the basis of the feedback loop: did the treatment achieve the goals? If it did, that's great. If it didn't, then a whole new line of thinking needs to be pursued:

- Is it possible that the diagnosis was wrong?
  - If the diagnosis is certain, what factors might account for the treatment failure?
- Are there things that the doctor or patient needs to do, which for some reason aren't happening, to help the treatment succeed? E.g., after knee surgery it's critical to get physical therapy. Without it, success rates are much lower.[342]
- Could a different treatment help?
  - What leads to the conclusion that a different treatment would be successful where the first one was not?
- And so forth.

Doctors and nurses would also need to capture whether the treatment *reduced* people's ability to lead the life they wanted in unexpected ways. That is, did the treatment cause side effects or other harm?

In summary, process improvement efforts related to feedback loops might involve creating ways to formalize treatment goals up front and then figure out if they have been met or not.

Deficiency

The big issue in health care is not a lack of money. It is what Dr. Don Berwick describes as "a deficiency of will and ambition,"[343] a failure to be serious about getting health care delivery to work better. The change that would make the biggest difference is to put the individual in the center of the equation.

CHAPTER THIRTEEN

The Blind Men and the Elephant

Twelve proposed solutions to the health care crisis are commonly discussed by lawmakers and policy makers. Many of these are excellent ideas, but all are likely to fail unless they are fit into this larger context: health care's focus needs to shift so that it is genuinely about you, with its goal being to enable people to lead the lives they want.

Fable

Four blind men are asked to describe an elephant. One touches its leg and says, "The elephant is like a tree trunk." The second touches its belly and says, "The elephant is like a wall." The third touches its ear and says, "The elephant is like a piece of cloth." The fourth grabs its tail and says, "The elephant is like a rope."[344] They were all correct, but they missed the larger picture.

Necessary but Not Sufficient

Proposals to fix health care in America have something in common with that story. Many of them are very insightful, but they all miss the larger picture. A number of them are absolutely necessary, but collectively they are not sufficient to move the dial.[345] They cannot live up to their promise unless health care focuses on a new, individual-centric purpose.

The twelve solutions discussed are:

- *UNIVERSAL COVERAGE* (Everyone has health insurance)
- *SINGLE PAYER* (The government pays directly for health care for everyone)
- *REGULATION* (Restrictions are imposed on the relationships between companies that make health products and the doctors and hospitals that use them)
- *COST CONTROLS* (Medicare, the federal health program for the elderly and disabled, cuts the prices it pays)
- *HEALTH INFORMATION TECHNOLOGY* (HIT) (Through electronic medical records and artificial intelligence, care is managed more efficiently and effectively)

- *COMPARATIVE EFFECTIVENESS* (An impartial organization researches and reports which treatments work better than others)
- *TRANSPARENCY* (Information about quality and cost of care is broadly available)
- *CONSUMER-DIRECTED HEALTH PLANS* (CDHP) (Consumers are better health care shoppers because they have a financial incentive to pay attention to cost and quality)
- *PAY FOR PERFORMANCE* (P4P) (Doctors are paid more if they deliver better care and less if they deliver worse care)
- *FOCUSED CARE* (Care providers are organized according to treatment or disease, and they compete on delivering the best outcomes for those)
- *ACCOUNTABLE CARE ORGANIZATIONS* (Multiple doctors and one or more hospitals voluntarily collaborate and are jointly responsible for costs and quality of care for a specified group of people)
- *MEDICAL HOME* (Primary care doctors coordinate all the needed care for their patients)

Each of the twelve topics is discussed briefly below. For the sake of simplicity it is assumed that each of these could actually be implemented as intended.

Universal Coverage

The premise: everyone should have health insurance, including the 47 million who are uninsured today.[346] Insurance may come from an employer, from the government, or be purchased privately, but no one should be without coverage. Various subsidies and safety nets are suggested to make coverage possible for people who couldn't otherwise afford it. Universal coverage is an excellent idea.

The limitations:

- The same quality issues that the health care system has today would affect more people. If more people had ready access to health care, fewer people would die due to under treatment — but more people would die due to medical errors and other side effects and complications.[347]
- There aren't enough doctors and nurses to treat a lot more people — not with the same approaches being used to treat people today.

Single Payer

The premise: the U.S. could save a lot of money — $128 billion a year by one estimate[348] — if we did what many other developed countries do and just had the government pay for health care for everyone.

The limitations: the same as those for Universal Coverage, above. Even assuming that this move fixed some of the *money* issues, it wouldn't fix health care *quality*.

Regulation

The premise: sometimes relationships are too cozy between doctors and hospitals, or between doctors/hospitals and manufacturers of drugs or medical products used in surgery. As a result, sometimes doctors may deliver care that makes money for them and for the hospital and/or manufacturer — while not necessarily being in the best interests of the patient.[349]

Prohibiting, regulating, or requiring reporting of those relationships — and how much doctors are paid as a result — is intended to get doctors to stop making decisions that profit them but may hurt patients.

The limitations: doctors are usually fairly quick to figure out new rules. The government has created many of them over the last several decades. Doctors adapt to preserve their income. Without addressing the underlying mindset — that health care is not individual-centric and needs to be — this behavior is unlikely to change.

Cost Controls

The premise: the government pays nearly half the costs of health care. It should use its purchasing power to negotiate lower prices.

The limitations: this approach has a track record of failure.[350] Two examples follow.

First, Medicaid, the shared federal and state health care program for poor people, has long required that it be given the lowest price that suppliers charge any customer. However, there were always exceptions.

One of those exceptions involved sales of contraceptives to college student health clinics. Historically, they were sold to the clinics for a fraction of their regular retail price. Those sales weren't included in the "lowest price" calculation.

That situation changed in 2007. If manufacturers had kept selling contraceptives for just a few dollars to student health clinics, they would have had to lower the price that they charged Medicaid. Instead, they doubled or quadrupled their prices to the student health clinics. That way they could keep the Medicaid price as it was.[351]

This attempt at cost control did not reduce Medicaid's costs. Instead it meant that a lot of college students could no longer afford birth control. Those results don't sound like an improvement from any angle.

Second, when Medicare (the federal health program for the elderly and disabled) cuts the rates it pays to doctors, the doctors start doing a lot more procedures. That way they don't see a drop in income. Said another way, the government doesn't end up spending less in total, even though it's paying less for each procedure. Instead more patients end up getting more tests and treatments.[352]

Given all of the problems discussed in previous chapters, you might guess that this effort at cost control probably has the unintended consequence of making many people's health worse.

Health Information Technology

The premise: lives and money can be saved by using EMR/EHR (Electronic Medical Records/Electronic Health Records); CPOE (Computerized Physician Order Entry — meaning that doctors' orders are electronic rather than handwritten); artificial intelligence; and other computerized aids to help with making decisions, managing and coordinating care, and keeping records.

A patient's entire health history could be available anytime, anywhere. Smart computer systems could help come up with an accurate diagnosis and could identify treatment options that took the individual's unique characteristics into account.

HIT (Health Information Technology) is an excellent idea, and would bring your health information up to the level of record-keeping that your supermarket has been using for decades to track how many cans of soup it sells.

The limitations:

- As noted in Chapter Seven, many doctors want to keep individuals from having access to much of the most critical information in their EMR/EHR. Unless this perspective changes, electronic records will fail to help individuals be better CEOs of their own health and health care.
- Unless health care changes its focus to be *to enable people to lead the lives they want*, all of those electronic records could simply end up documenting a high volume of acute interventions that don't improve people's lives. For example, consider the high volume of prostate testing and treatment, which in many cases may cause more harm than good. (This example is discussed in Chapter Twelve.)

Comparative Effectiveness

The premise: an impartial body evaluates the treatments for any given disease to determine which ones work best. Armed with this information, individuals and their doctors select treatments that are more likely to get good results, avoiding care that is known to get worse outcomes. A focus on comparative effectiveness is long overdue, so this is a great step forward.

The limitations: first, doctors tend to ignore the results of comparative effectiveness studies. For example, a big study in 2002 concluded that "generic pills for high blood pressure, which had been in use since the 1950s and cost only pennies a day, worked better than newer drugs that were up to 20 times as expensive." However, six years later, doctors' prescribing practices had barely budged.[353]

Second, patients behave in a similar way: "When it comes to comparative effectiveness, the track record of the American public and their doctors is not encouraging. Even when such comparisons are available, we tend to ignore them. . . . Whether it's invasive back surgery, medical scans or expensive drugs, patients and doctors alike often refuse to believe that costly treatments aren't worth it."[354]

Said another way, patients and doctors alike act as if the purpose of health care is to deliver acute interventions.

Third, as discussed previously, misdiagnosis is common and receives scant attention. As a result of comparative effectiveness, you might get an excellent treatment for a disease you don't have.

Fourth, most comparative effectiveness research focuses on clinical outcomes such as lowering blood pressure. It doesn't typically ask what the impact of a treatment is on people's ability to do the things they care about.

Transparency

The premise: "If you build it, they will come." That is, if information about quality and cost of care is broadly available, people will use it to make better health care decisions.

The limitations: this framework entirely ignores the fact that individuals are at a huge power disadvantage, have limited knowledge about how health care works, may be kept in the dark about their own health, and so forth. Because of these issues, people frequently don't have any meaningful way to use cost and quality information. In fact, research shows that people typically *don't* use this data when it is available to them[355] — which should come as no surprise.

Consumer-Directed Health Plans

The premise: high-deductible health insurance plans will encourage consumers to be better health care shoppers. Said another way, they have to pay more of their own money for health care before insurance kicks in, so they'll be more careful about spending it.

The limitations: first, language has been hijacked by marketers — since when does charging people more money make something "consumer-directed?"

Second, the math simply doesn't support this idea. Just 5% of the people use up 50% of the dollars spent on health care. And 20% of the people use up 80% of the health care dollars.[356] These numbers mean that the people whose care costs the most will probably blow by their high deductible in something like half a day's stay in the hospital. Thus, any incentive that having their money at risk is supposed to create is gone.

Third, the same objections discussed under Transparency, above, are issues here. In general it's wildly unrealistic to think that people can make objective analytical decisions about which doctors or hospitals to use and which tests and treatments to have, when they are kept so thoroughly uninformed about their own health and health care.

It's not possible to empower people by saying "You're empowered," when in a hundred ways their encounters with the health care system make it clear that they are not. Recall the example in Chapter Nine of the father who was fired by his child's doctor for asking questions. As one surgeon commented: "Who comes up with this stuff? Any plan that relies on the sheep to negotiate with the wolves is doomed to failure."[357]

Pay for Performance

The premise: the current payment model, in which doctors get paid just for doing things — regardless of whether they help or not — is not effective. Paying doctors and hospitals for following best practices, or for the outcomes of the care they deliver, will get them to do the right thing.

For example, the performance of hospitals and surgeons is measured on whether people get antibiotics in the 60 minutes before surgery, to prevent surgical infections. The performance of doctors is measured on whether people they treat who have diabetes have had their blood sugar levels checked with the most useful test at least once in the past twelve months.

The limitations: the measures that determine how much doctors get paid make little reference to the experience of the patient. Virtually all of the measures reflect traditional ideas of quality in health care. The measures evaluate:

- structure (e.g., "Do you transmit prescriptions electronically?")
- process (e.g., "For what percentage of your heart attack patients did you prescribe beta blockers?")
- outcomes (e.g., "What percentage of the patients you operated on had to be readmitted to the hospital within 30 days due to complications?")[358]

These focus primarily on the physicians' delivery of acute interventions. In some cases, patients are surveyed to determine how satisfied they are with the care they received. However, it is rare to find Pay for Performance measurement systems that track what percentage of the time the doctor:

- sought to discover the life priorities of people with chronic diseases
- explained the pros and cons of different treatments using consumer-friendly decision aids
- assisted individuals in selecting the treatment that best fit their values and preferences
- gave individuals their test results the day they were first available
- confirmed that individuals could repeat the name of the drug prescribed, the reason for taking it, and the dosing
- confirmed — not too long after prescribing a drug to someone with a chronic disease — that the drug was doing more good than harm

As a result of the types of activities that are tracked and rewarded and the types of activities that are not, Pay for Performance may not support the goal of making health care truly individual-centric.

Focused Care

The premise: "focused factories," an idea discussed by Regina Herzlinger of Harvard,[359] takes a very effective manufacturing concept and applies it to health care delivery. The premise is that it is hopelessly inefficient for individual doctors and hospitals to try to address the full range of health care issues from broken bones to brain surgery. Focusing instead on being spectacularly good at one thing — hernia repair or cataract surgery, for example — can yield huge quality and cost improvements.

Michael Porter, also of Harvard, and Elizabeth Teisberg, at the University of Virginia, suggest a concept which seems to me to be related to the "focused factories" framework. They propose that doctors self-organize into groups that focus on one disease and compete with other groups on the results that they can deliver.[360]

For instance, they might compete on lowering the percentage of people with asthma who end up in the emergency room, or on reducing the percentage of people with diabetes who have to have a limb amputated. The integration of care and the focus on results in terms that mean something to the people being treated are welcome features.

These are both constructive ideas.

The limitations: The focus is still largely on improving acute interventions, which is not always the same as helping people achieve the best health possible. In addition, many people have more than one medical condition. They can't be neatly divided up into disease buckets.

These solutions, like the others discussed, tend to omit the individual from the equation. Focused factories may not consider whether all of those acute interventions are beneficial to the patients, no matter how well they are done.

Porter and Teisberg's framework seems to imply that diseases can be treated almost independently from the person who has them. What if you have diabetes and depression and you get pregnant? How is your care coordinated then if depression and pregnancy aren't viewed as being within the scope of diabetes care? What happens if you have four or five major health problems, as the highest-cost patients do?[361]

What about the many issues that cut across health care, such as ICU Psychosis or the fact that people lack ready access to their own medical information?

Accountable Care Organizations

The premise: certain primary care doctors, specialists, and one or more hospitals work together to improve quality and cost of care for a specific group of patients such as elderly people on Medicare. They get paid based on the quality of care they deliver and on how efficiently they provide it. That is, the less they spend while getting excellent results, the better.

This concept is an attempt to get the benefits of integrated, coordinated care providers such as the Mayo Clinic (where the doctors are all on salary and electronic patient records are instantly available to all the other doctors) without requiring all the players to belong to one legal entity.

The limitations: again, one has to ask how quality of care is being defined. Is the definition based on the goal *to enable people to lead the lives they want?* Or does it instead reflect traditional measures of quality in health care — based on the framework of structure, process, and outcomes described above in Pay for Performance?

Medical Home

The premise: a team of professionals led by a primary care doctor and including nurses, administrative staff, and others, coordinate all the needed care for their patients.

While the concept behind primary care doctors has always been to coordinate care for their patients, in practice care has typically not been coordinated much at all. Consequences for individuals have often been devastating.

The new efforts to really, truly have primary care doctors coordinate care are a big improvement. Some of the features of medical homes are:

- having clearly defined processes for everything from scheduling appointments to reporting test results to individuals
- using Electronic Medical Records
- coordinating with specialists, hospitals, and other providers of tests and treatments
- coaching people to better manage their own health
- tracking to ensure that preventive care is given, that chronic conditions are managed, and that the team does what it says it will do[362]

These are all huge, huge wins. Doctors' offices that follow the guidelines for medical homes will give people much more information and help than is typical today, and will treat them with more consideration. These are great advantages.

The limitations: this effort is partly an attempt to shore up the dying field of primary care medicine. Recall that only 2% of medical students want to go into primary care. The concept of a medical home — with increased compensation for the coordinating work — elevates the importance of primary care.

However, it's not clear that putting one doctor in charge does enough to move the focus of health care from doctors to you. Primary care doctors are notoriously reluctant to challenge specialists. It's possible that an individual now might find the primary care doctor insisting on a particular treatment at a specialist's urging. That situation could put even more distance between the individual and answers to questions about the value and risks of the treatment.

Guidelines for medical homes[363] do not cover topics such as: improving the speed and accuracy of diagnosis; helping people address the meaning and impact of a major disease; helping them select treatments based on their priorities and values; and evaluating treatments to ensure that side effects are not swamping the benefits. All of these are necessary *to enable people to lead the lives they want.*

In the end, the ultimate medical home shouldn't be the primary care doctor's office. It should be you, wherever you are — twenty-four hours a day, seven days a week. It's your life. To get the best outcomes, you should be the locus of attention.

CHAPTER FOURTEEN

The Path Forward

Three changes are needed for health care to enable people to lead the lives they want. *The first is a social revolution that changes how the health care system regards the people it serves. The second is more realistic expectations about what health care can deliver. The third is management of health care as a process.*

Revolution

What's required to make health care individual-centric is a social revolution on the order of the one that freed the slaves or the one that gave women the vote. Before those two social revolutions, people with power made critical decisions for and had control over what happened to those two under-classes: women and slaves.

One justification given was the dubious notion that women and slaves didn't have the mental capacity— or interest in complex matters — necessary to be in charge of their own lives. Women and slaves were severely discounted and their concerns marginalized.

Individuals — patients — are in a very similar situation today. This revolution will make it unacceptable for the health care system to treat patients as second-class citizens whose intelligence, priorities, values, and needs can be safely ignored.

It would be possible to spend the next hundred years trying to work through each type of failure of health care to treat individuals as if their priorities and their lives counted. For example, a campaign could be launched to get the lights dimmed at night in ICUs to help stave off ICU Psychosis. The campaign that's been running *for over 160 years* to try to get doctors to wash their hands could be continued. And so forth.

But time is running out. Too many people are dying, and the health care system is on the verge of collapsing under its own weight.

People who receive care are severely discounted. Dealing with the symptoms of this fact is like campaigning to upgrade the shacks that slaves lived in from dirt floors to wood floors. Would that save lives? Sure. Was that the solution to the slaves' condition? Not by a mile.

The problem with slavery was *not* that slaves lived in shacks with dirt floors. The problem with slavery was *not* that slaves lived in shacks. The problem with slavery was the underlying mindset that made it acceptable to those with power that there were slaves at all.

The problem with health care is *not* that it hurts people nearly as often as it helps them. The problem with health care is *not* that it causes 26% of the deaths in this country. The problem with health care is that individuals are viewed with so little regard that conditions like these are not seen as urgent crises that demand immediate and massive attention — like the economic meltdown on Wall Street.

How else can you account for situations like those discussed in Chapter Four? For instance, good people in charge dismiss as *unimportant* the fact that the environment they create for individuals in an ICU drives a third of them clinically insane in as little as 24 hours. There's no way to explain that except by recognizing that people who seek help from the health care system are as discounted and marginalized as women and slaves were.

Seat Belts

Thirty years ago people rarely wore seat belts, drunk driving was common, and you couldn't see to the other side of any college classroom — it had disappeared under a thick haze of cigarette smoke.

Today most people wear seat belts, drunk driving is viewed as irresponsible, and more and more sites are declaring themselves smoke-free. While some of the mechanisms differ, efforts toward all of these changes have one thing in common: they make it clear that bad outcomes in these areas are not unavoidable.

They're not acts of God, something no one can do anything about. They're not just unfortunate-but-inevitable side effects of living. Instead, bad outcomes are a direct result of *choices* people make. The same is true in health care.

Medical errors, hospital-acquired infections, blood clots, and adverse drug events are not acts of God. Neither is the over use of many kinds of treatments or the failure to deliver basic preventive services. Nor is the failure to tell people the results of their medical tests. Nor is making health care inconvenient to get by insisting that people make weekday office visits when they could as easily get their needs addressed by e-mail.

These are all largely the result of *choices* that people involved in health care make. They have the option of making other choices.

What's required is a social revolution to change unspoken assumptions and attitudes, so that your needs are taken seriously.

Realistic Expectations

The second change needed for health care *to enable people to lead the lives they want* is for all of us to develop more realistic expectations about what health care can and should deliver. Two issues result from ceding so much power and control to the health care system:

- First, people place themselves at the complete mercy of a very flawed system that has repeatedly demonstrated that it can harm people nearly as often as it helps them.
- Second, it is not reasonable to expect the health care system by itself to fix problems that people help create through their own behavior.

Sawdust and Planks

Faced with the facts discussed in this book so far, how can you not be outraged? But here's something to think about: most of us aren't completely meticulous about nailing every detail, either. For example, fewer than 10% of us actually follow these basic recommendations:

- eat 5 servings of fruit and vegetables daily
- exercise for 30 minutes 4-5 times a week
- drink moderately
- don't smoke[364]

Comic strips, always a great reflection of the culture, add insight. Here is the dialog from a Hagar the Horrible comic:

Hagar: "My doctor said I have to make big changes in my diet. . . . He said I have to switch from beer to water . . . and switch from fatty foods to fresh vegetables!"

Lucky Eddie: "Wow! What are you going to do?"

Hagar: "I'm going to switch doctors."[365]

We're expecting doctors to fix us up regardless of what we do.

Consider those hospital-acquired infections once again. When the numbers are calculated, it turns out that people pick up measurable infections in hospitals probably in less than one in a thousand encounters, and those infections cause deaths in less than one out of every twenty-two thousand encounters.[366]

That's no excuse for the infections, and no comfort at all to anyone who's been seriously injured or watched a family member die from one of these infections. What it does mean, though, is that it's not very reasonable to assume that the rest of us would do any better. The percentage of people who don't always wash their hands has been increasing:

- 15% don't wash after using the toilet
- 35% don't wash before lunch
- 39% don't wash after sneezing[367]

You may be spreading infections if you visit someone in the hospital. You put your unwashed hand on the doorknob . . . then on the soda or coffee machine, the elevator buttons, the counters. If the next people who come along are doctors or nurses, they'll pick up whatever bugs you transmitted, and they'll very efficiently pass them along to the next patient they see if they don't wash their hands.

If you're carrying nasty germs — or pick some up on your way to the patient room you are visiting — and then touch the guard rails on the bed, the blanket, the doorknob to the bathroom, the faucets on the sink, anything else in the room, and/or the patient, you could easily be the direct source of an infection that the patient picks up.

On a similar note, responsibility for some adverse drug events can be traced to patients who don't follow dosing instructions. For example, they may double up on doses and end up overdosing themselves. They may "borrow" drugs from other people — drugs that are inappropriate for them. They may start or stop taking medicines abruptly when the drug dose needs to be ramped up or tapered off slowly.

They may decide on their own to take a mix of current prescription drugs, old prescriptions drugs left over from a previous illness, and over-the-counter drugs — creating a stew of conflicting chemicals in their bloodstreams.

In other words, the responsibility for some of the illnesses and deaths that result from care delivery can be laid directly at the feet of patients and their families. Individuals are part of the health care delivery system even if this fact is not generally acknowledged.

Both patients and doctors are exasperated that the other group doesn't do what it's supposed to. Doctors can point to the fact that one study forecasts a drop of five years in life expectancy in the U.S.[368] due to the rise in obesity and consequent complications of diabetes, widely viewed as resulting from the failure of individuals to do the right things regarding diet and exercise.[369]

They might point to the fact that the CDC (Centers for Disease Control and Prevention) has concluded that "80% of diabetes, heart disease, and stroke could be eliminated through reductions in smoking and obesity."[370] They might say, "If people aren't going to make the effort to help themselves, why complain about what we do when we try to fix what they've done wrong?"

Individuals can point to the fact that about 26% of all deaths in this country are directly caused by health care, as discussed in Chapter One.

One is reminded of the biblical quotation, "Why do you look at the speck of sawdust in your brother's eye and pay no attention to the plank in your own eye?"[371] Said another way, it's a reminder to everyone to clean up their own act before objecting to other people's shortcomings. Maybe we need to rethink our expectation that doctors should be much more consistent and deliberate guardians of our health than we are.

The Fisherman and His Wife

In the fairy tale the fisherman's wife demands that he petition a magic fish (who is really an enchanted prince) for ever grander homes and loftier positions — king, emperor, and Lord. Each wish is granted, until the final one: she has gone too far, and the fisherman comes home to find her living in the hovel in which they started.

In health care, we petition the enchanted princes — the doctors — to save us. But we may have gone too far. Americans consume a staggering amount of resources to get health care:

- One out of ten employed civilians work in health care.[372]
- Health care spending in the U.S. averages $8,160 per person per year.[373]
- More than sixteen cents out of every dollar in the U.S. economy goes into health care.[374]

Most economists, business leaders, government officials, and health policy experts think that this level of spending on health care — and continued rapid growth in health care costs projected in the coming years — is more than the country can afford. Every dollar spent on health care means one less dollar to spend on schools, roads, housing, and other important services or objects.

We have developed unrealistic expectations that doctors and the U.S. economy can't possibly meet. We are on the brink of seeing the health care system implode of its own excesses, restoring us to the metaphorical hovel in which we started: dramatically limited availability of health care.

It might be constructive to put a little less faith in the enchanted princes' ability to solve all of our health problems like magic, and start asking what we could do differently ourselves. Perhaps we've accidentally replaced a desire for *good health* with a desire for *acute interventions.*

Here's what one business leader, Paul Otellini, had to say: "From the 19th-century birth of clinics, medical technologies and specialty care, we have inherited two fundamental assumptions that no longer serve us well in the 21st century: 1) We wait for an illness or injury; 2) then we travel to a medical institution for an expert to repair things. We centralize infrastructure and expertise in ever larger urban hospitals and clinics that have become marble and steel monuments to medicine."[375]

He continued: "With the large number of uninsured and underinsured in America and our staggering $2.4 trillion health care bill, we can no longer afford this pilgrimage to expensive and crowded medical centers for our every health care need. Nor can we relinquish all responsibility for our well-being to the doctors and caregivers who perform miracles every day to put us back together again."[376]

Stress Out

Why do people do things that are bad for their health? Research into stress provides some clues. One study notes: "People who are chronically exposed to psychologically stressful environments over-consume calorie-rich foods."[377] It goes on to say: "The study is an advance in understanding the psychological basis for the sharp increase in obesity across all age groups since the mid-1970s."[378]

Other experts concur. For example, the Mayo Clinic notes: "When you're under stress, you may find it harder to keep up healthy-eating habits. Also, during particularly stressful times, you may eat in an attempt to fulfill emotional needs, which is sometimes called stress eating. And you may be especially likely to eat high-calorie foods during times of stress, even when you're not hungry. To combat weight problems during stress and reduce the risk of obesity, you need to get a handle on your stress."[379]

Stress can lead to increased smoking and drug and alcohol abuse. It can also cause a lack of focus and other unwanted mental and emotional conditions, as well as other ills such as heart disease and back pain.[380]

Couple that picture with research about the health of baby boomers, reported in an article titled, "Baby Boomers Appear To Be Less Healthy Than Parents." It notes that "a growing body of evidence suggests that they may be the first generation to enter their golden years in worse health than their parents."[381]

It goes on to say: "They are more likely to report difficulty climbing stairs, getting up from a chair and doing other routine activities, as well as more chronic problems such as high cholesterol, blood pressure and diabetes. . . . Boomers tend to report more stress than earlier generations — from their jobs, their commutes, taking care of their parents and their kids — all of which can take a physical toll."[382]

Now What?

Stress drives people to self-destructive behavior, stress creates medical problems, and stress levels are soaring. Recall that the CDC estimates that up to 90% of doctors' visits have stress at their root.[383]

One article noted that "Americans eat worse, exercise less and count on pills and doctors to bail them out more than the residents of any other country."[384] If you decide that you want to change this picture for yourself, one place to start might be to consider how to manage the stress you feel.[385]

What are your options? There are countless suggestions for you from television, newspapers and magazines, the internet, your employer, and your insurance company. Rather than repeating any of that advice, what follows is a possibility that may be under-represented in those sources. It involves a practical, insightful way to clarify your priorities.

Priorities

One way to reduce stress is to think through whether you are putting your time into things that you value or not, and if not, what choices you have to change the situation.

Stephanie Winston has written an unusually useful book, *Getting Out From Under: Redefining Your Priorities in an Overwhelming World*.[386] She offers a series of exercises so simple that they seem almost hokey, and one is tempted to dismiss them as unlikely to tell you anything you don't already know.

However, actually *doing* the exercises can yield surprising insights about what genuinely matters to you and what doesn't. Those insights can lead you to reconsider the commitments you make and how they contribute — or fail to contribute — to your satisfaction with your life.

Creating a better fit between what you genuinely value and where you spend your time can reduce stress and may make it easier for you to make choices that improve your health and enable you to lead the life you want.

On a similar note, a research study showed that "when people invested more in intrinsic values, like relationships and quality of life, and less in consumption, it seemed to increase their happiness. . . . The three main intrinsic values were being connected to family and friends, exploring one's interests or skills and 'making the world a better place.'"[387]

The Third Leg of the Stool

The first two changes needed to address the health care crisis, described above, are:

- *A social revolution* that makes it unacceptable to treat people who seek help from the health care system as second-class citizens whose priorities don't count.
- *More realistic expectations* about what the health care system can do. It cannot eliminate death or fix every health problem that people help create through their own behavior.

The third change needed is *management of health care as a process*. As discussed in Chapter Eleven and in Chapter Twelve, failures to clarify the purpose of health care and to manage all the steps in the process of care in a coordinated way result in a lot of activity that delivers no benefit. The first two steps — social revolution and more realistic expectations — will not, by themselves, solve the health care crisis.

A process that is not managed in a coordinated way may be described as "fragmented." Here is what one foundation working to improve health care says:

"The fragmentation of our delivery system is a fundamental contributor to the poor overall performance of the U.S. health care system. In our fragmented system:

- Patients and families navigate unassisted across different providers and care settings, fostering frustrating and dangerous patient experiences;
- Poor communication and lack of clear accountability for a patient among multiple providers lead to medical errors, waste, and duplication;
- The absence of peer accountability, quality improvement infrastructure, and clinical information systems foster poor overall quality of care; and
- High-cost, intensive medical intervention is rewarded over higher-value primary care, including preventive medicine and the management of chronic illness."[388]

In other words, health care isn't being managed with an eye towards getting you optimal outcomes; it's run as an uncoordinated collection of activities, the outcome of which is highly variable and almost random: sometimes great, sometimes tragic. If health care is genuinely going to be about you, it needs to be managed as a process.

That process management needs to include you as a key player. Recall the situation described in Chapter Three in which low-income parents cut trips to the emergency room by half once they were taught how to use thermometers and other basic skills. The fact that the health care system hasn't jumped on this win and copied it across the country is due to the fact that patients and their families aren't typically considered part of the process of health care.

That perspective needs to change. It's not possible to successfully run a process involving your health without including you.

CHAPTER FIFTEEN

Surviving the Geeks-in-Garages Era

Thirty years ago, only geeks had personal computers. They built them in their garages. Today four-year-olds use personal computers. Health care today is where personal computers were thirty years ago: not easy to work with or to get what you need from. As health care works its way through the geeks-in-garages era to a better future, you can take steps to get better results today.

Punch Cards

Forty years ago — before the geeks-in-garages era — if you wanted to do any computer work, your experience might have looked like this:

First you had to learn a computer language, probably one called FORTRAN or COBOL. These were taught in semester-long college courses, and one semester certainly didn't make you an expert.

After painstakingly learning arcane programming rules, you wrote your program and recorded it on punch cards — pieces of thin cardboard about the thickness of a file folder and about three inches high and seven inches long.[389] Each punch card probably held the equivalent of less than a sentence. You carefully rubber-banded the stack of cards and dropped them off at the data center.

The serious computing — the institutional computing — was done during normal business hours. Running programs for amateurs like you was relegated to the wee hours of the morning. You would pick up the results of the run of your program from the rack outside the data center the next day.

If you'd made a tiny mistake in your program — misplaced a comma, say — the result would be garbage. Then you'd have to correct your punch cards, submit them the following night, and wait for the results to be ready the day after that. Thus, it could easily take you days to get meaningful output from a ten-line program.

People who were going to make a career of programming were generally the only ones who continued to study to learn its nuances. The work *you* produced was roughly equivalent to a young child's arts and crafts project.

The data center people were very powerful. They controlled access to computers. No computing happened unless they agreed to do it. There was no such thing as a personal computer, so programs like e-mail, Word for word processing, Excel for spreadsheets, and Quicken for tracking your finances had not been invented yet.

Fanatics

Ten years after that — thirty years ago — just about everyone was still at the mercy of the data centers. Most computing was done by trained experts whose professional lives were completely focused on mainframe (big computer) computing.

Only hard-core fanatics on the fringe had personal computers. They built them by hand. They were just starting to break the traditional experts' stranglehold on computing, and the experts fought back vigorously.

If you'd suggested even to the personal computer fanatics that one day four-year-olds would use PCs, they'd have snorted in derision at your obvious naiveté about the incredible complexities that only they could master.

Today health care is where personal computers were thirty years ago.[390] Only people who are nearly as fanatical about their health as computer geeks were about personal computing typically wrest the best outcomes from the health care system.

If health care were designed *to enable people to lead the lives they want*, it would be nearly as easy for you to understand how to achieve the best health possible as it is for four-year-olds to use personal computers. Health and health care would not be viewed as the exclusive territory of the experts who today exert so much control.

Before a hue and cry is raised about shifting some health care capability out of the experts' realm and into individuals' hands — Would you perform brain surgery on yourself?! — note that of course many health care tasks will still require highly trained experts, as do many computing tasks today.

But there's an enormous amount of computer work that you and I can do today, given a personal computer and programs *created by experts* for e-mail, word processing, spreadsheets, presentations, and so forth. And there should be an enormous amount that you and I can do about our health without having to interact face-to-face with a highly trained health care expert.

Marcus Welby, Redux

What about the people who don't want to have anything to do with their health and health care? What about the people who still just want Marcus Welby, M.D. to take care of everything? Three answers follow:

First, some people don't want to deal with managing their health and health care because it's too hard, too complicated, and too confusing. For those people, making it easier would . . . make it easier.

They might find that they would be more interested if it weren't so bewildering — if they could understand clearly what to do and how to do it; if they had the information to make good decisions; and if actions taken by the health care system were coordinated and led to better outcomes. Thus, the percentage of people who elected not to engage would be likely to drop.

Second, whether any of us likes it or not, the people who pay for health care will increasingly be encouraging us to get involved. They know that our health depends to a large degree on what we personally do, not on what doctors do.

They want us to be healthy — partly because they need to have productive employees or citizens, and partly because sickness is so expensive. We'll increasingly face incentives — and big costs if we don't get involved in our own health and health care.

Third, there will always be some people who don't engage, even if health and health care are made a lot simpler. Then what? Well, the fact that *others* don't engage doesn't mean that *you* shouldn't. And it means that the health care system needs to work even harder to make health care even simpler to deal with so that engaging will be more appealing.

The hard fact is that those who don't engage are likely to suffer poorer health and higher expenses than they would if they did engage. The data's already in on that one.

Tool Kit

How do you thrive in this era of health care? Make use of the following tool kit:

- understand your responsibilities as CEO of your own health and health care
- recognize questions to consider in your role as CEO
- know what danger spots to watch out for, especially concerning:
  - diagnosis
  - treatment options
  - care delivery (e.g., surgery)
  - post-treatment management

- identify resources you can draw on, such as:
  - quality and cost comparison websites
  - checklists and decision aids, covering topics such as:
    - visiting the doctor
    - choosing a treatment
    - being in the hospital
- learn common, potentially fatal assumptions to watch out for

Each of these is discussed in more detail below.

CEO Responsibilities

Three things you can do to improve the odds that you will get the benefits of modern medicine without so many of the dangers and downsides are:

1. Ask questions.
2. Keep a Personal Health Record.
3. Learn how the health care system works, especially where things tend to go wrong.

Ask Questions

When you plan to see a doctor, it's an excellent idea to come prepared with two copies of a list of the questions you have, one for you and one for the doctor. You can, of course, create your own list from scratch. However, if you want to jump-start your efforts, one interactive website that can be useful is called Question Builder. It can be found at http://www.ahrq.gov/questionsaretheanswer/questionbuilder.aspx.

The website offers about a dozen different questions you might ask in each of nine different situations:

1. Receiving a prescription
2. Being prescribed a medical test
3. Receiving a diagnosis
4. Considering treatment options
5. Considering surgery
6. Choosing a health insurance plan
7. Choosing a doctor or other care provider
8. Choosing a hospital
9. Choosing a long-term care facility (that is, a nursing home)

Examples of questions suggested when you are considering treatment are:

- How soon do I need to make a decision about treatment?
- What happens if I choose to have no treatment at all?

The site allows you to select and print out just the questions that you want to address.

Keep a Personal Health Record

A PHR (Personal Health Record) can save your life. It can also save you time, money, and aggravation. Until all your health records are instantly available electronically to you and to any doctor or hospital that might provide care to you, one of the most useful steps you can take to improve the care you get is to keep a PHR.

People often have limited information about their own medical history, and that can be dangerous. They don't know what tests they've had, what the results were, what conclusions the doctors have drawn, and so forth.

When they see different doctors over time, they can't clearly explain their medical history. They may undergo the same tests multiple times and experience unnecessary delays, risks, and costs.

Doctors often can't connect the dots because they don't have the whole story. As a result, people's health can suffer as they shuttle from one doctor to the next. For now, the only person in a position to fix that problem may be you. If you have your complete medical record you will be able to be a more active player in your own medical care and health management.

As used here, the term PHR implies a comprehensive record of your health information. It includes:

- information that comes from you, such as notes about symptoms you have
- information that comes from people or organizations that have tested or treated you (doctors, labs, and hospitals), such as medical test results and doctors' notes from office visits

One website that offers a perspective on PHRs is http://www.myphr.com.

The first step is to get a complete copy of your medical records, going back as many years as you think makes sense.

Georgetown University's Health Policy Center has an organization called the Center on Medical Records Rights and Privacy. It has created a brochure for each state that explains exactly how to go about getting your medical records. Each one is titled "Your Medical Record Rights in [name of state]." These can be downloaded free from http://ihcrp.georgetown.edu/privacy/records.html.

One decision for you to make is what type and format of PHR you want to keep. If you want to keep your record electronically, which is what most people recommend today, that implies either that you are able to get all of your medical records electronically or that you have a scanner and plan to scan them in to your computer.

You can see if your health insurance company or your primary care doctor's office offers its own PHR. Generally, this means that information is tracked on a secure website, with password-controlled access.

These may be good options, but recognize that over time your insurer and your doctor may change; it could be a problem if you were to lose access to your information if that happened. Additionally, PHRs provided by insurers or doctors may not allow you to record everything that you have decided you want to track.

Other options are PHRs provided by third parties not associated with your medical care. Two of these are Google Health, which can be found at http://www.google.com/intl/en-US/health/about/ and Microsoft HealthVault, at http://www.healthvault.com. Because PHRs are rapidly evolving, you may find other excellent options online if you search for "online personal health records."

It is also possible to find reviews that compare these two PHRs and others by searching online. You might search on: compare Google Health and Microsoft HealthVault. Reviews are not included here because PHR offerings are in a constant state of change and upgrade.

Other options include keeping your information on a flash drive or mobile phone so that it is portable. Searching on the term "portable PHR" is likely to lead to some feasible options.

Additionally, you might elect to keep your records on paper without any computers involved. One factor to consider is how comfortable you are with the privacy policies and data security of any computerized solution.

In addition to medical records from your doctors and other providers of tests and treatments, it's a good idea to include a record of every health encounter in your PHR. Examples of these are events such as a visit to a doctor, a dentist, or an eye care provider (whether a doctor or not); a flu shot at a local drugstore; a visit to other providers such as a chiropractor or acupuncturist; a medical test; a hospital stay; phone calls with any of the above people or organizations; or any other interaction with the health care system. Information to capture might include:

- complete contact information for the provider and/or facility
- why you contacted them
- what tests they ran
- what they said was wrong

- what they said to do
- any medicines prescribed, with the spelling of the name, the strength (e.g., 500 mg), dosing instructions (e.g., take 4 times a day with food), and duration (e.g., ten days)
- next steps:
  - what they are going to do
  - when you will hear back about test results
  - when you are supposed to come back or who else you are supposed to see, and so forth

It will also be useful to record significant symptoms and any other personal data that's relevant to your care. For example, some people will want to track their weight, exercise routine, and other similar facts.

Once you have created your PHR, it will make sense to take it with you (or print out and take relevant sections) when you go to see a doctor, enter the hospital, or have any other significant encounter with the health care system. Then you will be in a position to provide complete and accurate answers to questions about your medical history; to prevent expensive and potentially risky duplication of tests; to avoid being given treatments to which you previously had a bad reaction; and so forth.

Learn How the Health Care System Works

Your third responsibility as CEO of your own health and health care is to understand enough about how health care works so that you know what to do to get the best results you can. You have already come a long way in understanding what some of the weaknesses of the health care system are by reading this book. Here are four points to remember:

1. It typically isn't anyone's job in health care to ensure that you get the best outcomes. Their jobs are typically to run tests and deliver treatments. Right now it's largely up to you to think through what results are important to you and to make your way through the health care system in pursuit of those goals.
2. Doctors have many reasons for suggesting more treatment than you would want if you clearly understand the benefits and risks.
3. Health care today is not managed as a process: the steps in health care are not typically well-connected or linked together. It's often necessary for you to provide the linkages.
4. There are many, many opportunities for things to go wrong, and it's important to pay attention and ask questions if something doesn't seem right.

If you are interested in learning more about how health care works, here are five books/websites to consider:

1. *Guide to Health Care Quality: How to Know It When You See It* published by the federal Agency for Healthcare Research and Quality. This 20-page booklet is available for free download from http://www.ahrq.gov/consumer/guidetoq/guidetoq.pdf. Additionally, if you call the contact number listed on the web site they will even send you a hard copy at no charge. The booklet covers topics such as:

   - what is meant by quality in health care
   - how to avoid over treatment and under treatment
   - ways to monitor chronic conditions such as diabetes and heart disease
   - how to find information about the quality of hospitals, nursing homes, health plans, and doctors
   - questions to ask
   - websites that can provide more information

2. *You The Smart Patient: An Insider's Guide for Getting the Best Treatment* by Michael F. Roizen, Mehmet C. Oz, and The Joint Commission. Doctors Roizen and Oz have written many books about health care and Dr. Oz has appeared on *Oprah*. The Joint Commission inspects hospitals and says whether they are operating according to nationally recognized standards or not.

   The book's back jacket notes: "The book shows readers in clear, easy steps how to take control of their own health care and deal with all matters that may come up when facing a medical case: from choosing the right doctor, hospital, and insurance company to navigating prescription drugs, specialists, treatment options, alternative medicine, pain management, or any problem that might arise." The book is written with humor and it has a big advantage: it is easy to understand.

3. *Understanding Healthcare* by Richard Saul Wurman. This book has lots of pictures, charts, and diagrams and very clear, concise explanations answering questions like:

   - "How do the most popular diets compare?"
   - "What are the safety risks in using medicines?"
   - "What can I expect as I age?"
   - "How can I get the most out of a doctor's visit?"
   - "What do my test results mean?"
   - "What are my treatment options?"

- "What should I know about my doctor?"
- "What does an operating room look like?"
- "How do health plans work?"
- "What is Medicare?"

It provides lists of questions to ask about tests, illnesses, and treatments.

4. *How's Your Health?* by John Wasson and Regina Benjamin. This book is available for free download from www.howsyourhealth.org and uses an Alice in Wonderland theme to highlight some of the issues in health care. It focuses on how to solve health care problems that people often run into, from not understanding the risks they face to not being able to afford care.

The introduction has sections titled, "Doctor Time is Odd," "Doctor Language is Often Strange," and "Common Sense is Not So Very Common." The website includes opportunities to take a health survey and to create a Personal Health Record, and provides guidance on problem solving as well as suggestions for other websites to visit. For instance, it provides a link to the Mayo Clinic to check what your symptoms might mean.

5. *The Social Transformation of American Medicine: The Rise of a Sovereign Profession and the Making of a Vast Industry* by Paul Starr. This book won the Pulitzer Prize and its writing was an extraordinary feat. The book explains the history of doctors and health care from early Colonial America to the modern era.

Despite the fact that it was published in 1982, it provides an exceptionally fine explanation of how health care got to be the way it is today. While it's very comprehensible, it is a strategic analysis and does not get to the level of advising you how to address your medical needs.

CEO Questions

These questions are for you yourself:

- "What do I want from the health care system?"
  - If you go along with the idea that "health is the absence of abnormality,"[391] then you will need to be prepared to spend a lot of time and money with the health care system. Virtually everyone has many minor abnormalities which don't interfere with daily living.
  - If instead you choose a goal that's less about health care and more about you — e.g., to enable you to lead the life you want — you may find that it's easier to focus on what you genuinely need.

- "To what extent do I want to be involved in my own care and decisions?" Options might include:
  - I want to collect all the information and make all the decisions myself.
  - I want my family to help me decide.
  - I want to discuss the pros and cons of the different options with my doctor and then decide.
  - I want the doctor to decide.
- "How will I ensure that my care is coordinated if several different doctors, labs, hospitals, other professionals, and other organizations are involved in my care?"
  - You may discover that you yourself need to be the coordinator.

Danger Spots: Diagnosis

Some potential problems with the diagnostic process are:

1. You have tests that don't seem to serve any purpose.
2. You aren't ever told the results of tests.
3. You are told that a test says you *have* a certain disease, when you *don't*.
4. You are told that a test says you *don't have* a certain disease, when you *do*.
5. Your symptoms are a pretty close fit for a disease familiar to the doctor, so she doesn't consider other possibilities even though some of your symptoms don't fit.
6. You're told that you are fine because the tests didn't find anything, but you are pretty sure that you aren't fine.
7. You're so shocked by hearing that you have a serious problem that you can't think straight.

Each of these is discussed further below.

Tests With No Purpose

One year Julie's doctor sent her for a breathing test. The results were excellent. Her doctor then sent her to a pulmonary specialist, just to get a second opinion on some of the details in the results. When she arrived at the specialist's office, the staff started to set her up to do the same breathing test she'd just had.

When she objected that she had brought the very current results of the previous test with her and asked why she had to repeat the test, the answer was: "Every patient who walks through the door has to have this test before seeing the doctor."

When she protested this waste of time and money — this absence of any medical reason for the test — she was told that the appointment would be cancelled if she did not comply.

She went ahead with the test only because her primary care doctor was eager to get the specialist's opinion. The test produced the same excellent results as the previous one. She would not ever elect to go back to that doctor again.

Before you agree to a test, two questions to consider asking are:

- What will this test tell us that we don't already know?
- What will change in my treatment or health as a result of this test?

Both of these are variations on, "Is this test really necessary?" It is surprising how often the honest answer is no. If you get an answer like, "It is standard practice to order this test," that's a hint to think about finding another doctor.

Tests With No Report Out

This topic is discussed at length in Chapter Seven. When you agree to have a test, steps you can take to help ensure that you hear the results and have the documentation you need for your Personal Health Record include:

1. Ask the doctor for the *name of the test* and write it down.
2. Ask *when* you will be notified of the results, *by what medium* (phone, mail, e-mail, or some other way) and *by whom*.
3. Ask to have a copy of the actual test results mailed to you (not simply a postcard that says "Your test was fine.")
4. Make a note on your calendar of the date by which you should receive the results (or two notes, if you will receive a phone call first and a paper copy in the mail after that). If you haven't received them by then, call the doctor's office promptly.

False Positives and False Negatives

A false positive is a test result that says you have a disease you don't. A false negative is a test result that says you do not have a disease when you actually do. Michael Blastland and Andrew Dilnot explain surprising facts about these two problems, using mammograms for breast cancer as an example.[392] The discussion below is drawn from their work.

Assume that 8 women out of every 1000 who get mammograms actually have breast cancer. Assume further that the test will find 9 out of 10 breast cancers. And finally, assume that 7% of the time it will say that someone has breast cancer when she doesn't.

Out of 1,000 women, 7 of the 8 who have cancer will be told that they have cancer. The test will miss the eighth one. The other 992 women do not have cancer but 7% of them, or roughly 70 people, will be told that they do have cancer. So a total of 77 people will be told that they have breast cancer when in fact only 7 of them do. That means that only 1 of every 11 people told as a result of a mammogram that they have breast cancer actually do have cancer.[393]

The danger with false positives is that they can lead to a lot more testing and, in some cases, unnecessary treatment. People not familiar with statistics and health care tend to assume that if the test says you have a disease, then you have it. However, as the numbers above suggest, that is often far from the case.

A book that does a very good job of explaining the problems with taking test results and treatment plans at face value is *The Patient from Hell: How I Worked with My Doctors To Get the Best of Modern Medicine and How You Can Too* by Stephen H. Schneider, Ph.D. with Janica Lane.

The title is more provocative than accurate; what the author means is that he was determined to get the best care and consequently asked a lot of questions about assumptions his doctors were making about the tests they used and treatments they recommended. He discovered that these were often based on erroneous thinking or sloppy science.

Misdiagnosis

Misdiagnosis is so common that it pays to be on the lookout for it. *How Doctors Think* by Jerome Groopman provides great insight into this problem.

The cover blurb notes, "Dr. Jerome Groopman lifts the veil on possibly the most taboo topic in medicine: the pervasive nature of misdiagnosis. His engrossing narrative exposes all of the subtle mental traps — the snap judgments and stereotypical thinking, the premature conclusions and herd instinct — that dangerously narrow the vision of too many physicians."

Dr. Groopman suggests three questions to ask if you are uncertain that the diagnosis hits the mark:

1. "What else could it be?"
2. "Is there anything that doesn't fit?"
3. "Is it possible I have more than one problem?"[394]

"There's nothing wrong with you."

When you are told that you are fine when you are pretty sure that you are not, it is a challenge to figure out how to proceed.

Doctors distinguish between "signs," which are abnormalities they can see or measure — such as high blood pressure or low blood count — and "symptoms," which are things they can't see but that you experience. Pain is a symptom, for example. Doctors sometimes discount symptoms unless they can see corresponding signs.

One defense is to keep good records. That is, notice when the pain (or other symptom) occurs and what is going on when it does. Are you eating? Sleeping? Exercising? Working? Engaged in some other activity?

Track what you do to try to address the symptom and to what degree it helps. And so forth. This careful capture of data may help your doctor recognize what your problem is.

A web site that may be useful is the Mayo Clinic Symptom Checker, available at: http://mayoclinic.com/health/symptom-checker/DS00671.

Shock

When you are told that you have a serious medical problem, you may be so shocked that you can't think straight. That's entirely normal. The danger is that you may agree to further tests or treatments when you are in a daze and haven't had a chance to wrap your mind around the facts.

One defense is for you to take someone else with you to appointments that you suspect may involve troubling news, and ask them to take notes and ask questions if you can't — for example, "If we take a few days to absorb this information, will that cause any worsening of her health?"

An excellent resource is Jessie Gruman's book, *AfterShock: What to Do When the Doctor Gives You — or Someone You Love — a Devastating Diagnosis.* The book is packed with very practical suggestions from someone who has been diagnosed on four separate occasions with life-threatening illnesses. A few of the many topics she discusses are:

- common reactions to the shock
- common sense advice for getting through the first 48 hours
- deciding how much information you need about your disease and its treatment
- choosing what/how much to say to other people about your diagnosis, and how to involve family and friends
- finding the right doctors, hospitals, and expert opinions, including how to approach getting an appointment when doctors are booked for months in advance
- deciding how to deal with your employer
- working with your health insurer
- managing your own reactions over time and reducing stress as you proceed

Another fine book is Elise NeeDell Babcock's *When Life Becomes Precious: The Essential Guide for Patients, Loved Ones, and Friends of Those Facing Serious Illnesses.* While it is focused on cancer, its advice seems applicable to issues that may arise concerning virtually all serious diseases.

A few of the chapter titles are:

- "Eleven Common Reactions: Understanding Your Feelings"
- "Why We Stop Talking When We Need to Start: How Our Fears Divide Us"
- "What Do I Say?: How to Begin Talking When You Don't Know What to Say"
- "The One Who Needs You: Providing Comfort to the Primary Caregiver"
- "Sharing the News and Helping Children Understand When a Loved One is Ill"
- "Making Holidays Meaningful"

Both of these books are very readable and may lead you to feel as if you have a friend at hand who has a very clear sense of what you are going through.

Danger Spots: Treatment Options

Some of the dangers involved when doctors discuss treatment options with you are:

1. Creating the impression that you have to decide on the spot (unless you are in the emergency room, you usually have days, and sometimes weeks or months, to decide).
2. Creating the impression that you don't have a choice; that the decision is really theirs.
3. Telling you that there is only one solution.
4. Telling you about a number of solutions, but presenting the information in such a way that only one solution sounds good.
5. Not providing you with any written comparisons of the treatment options such as a chart listing the pros and cons of each option.
6. Not considering your priorities, values, and preferences in their recommendation.
7. Omitting data about what percentage of people are actually helped by the treatment.
8. Underplaying the risks of the option they recommend.

Three books that may help you remedy these shortcomings are:

1. *How Patients Should Think* by Ray Moynihan & Melissa Sweet. This book devotes a chapter to each of ten major questions, and at the end of each chapter additional related questions are offered. The overarching theme is to be skeptical of the assertions made to you. The ten major questions are:

    1. "Do I really need that test?"
    2. "Do I really have that disorder?"

3. "Do I really need to be screened?"
4. "What are my options?"
5. "How well does that treatment work?"
6. "What are the side effects?"
7. "Will this operation really help?"
8. "What is the evidence?"
9. "Who else is profiting here?"
10. "What can I do to help myself?"

2. *Worried Sick* by Nortin M. Hadler. Dr. Hadler has been raising the alarm for years about the fact that many tests and treatments help far fewer people than are given them, particularly if the people in question have only a minor illness or abnormality. This book dissects the science behind claims for a large number of tests and treatments and finds most of them wanting. One warning: this book is very well-researched but some people may find it a little hard to follow.

3. *My Mother, Your Mother: Embracing "Slow Medicine," the Compassionate Approach to Caring for Your Aging Loved Ones* by Dennis McCullough. Dr. McCullough makes a very compelling case for thinking twice before agreeing to aggressive tests or treatment of health problems in older people; those treatments often cause a lot more problems than they fix. It explains how to prepare for the inevitable health crises of the elderly and to help ensure that they are not damaged by the layering on of treatment after treatment in the heat of the emergency.

Danger Spots: Care Delivery

Many of the early chapters in this book identified problems with care delivery that takes place in a hospital. Three books that provide insight into hazards to watch out for are:

1. *How to Get Out of the Hospital Alive: A Guide to Patient Power* by Sheldon P. Blau and Elaine Fantle Shimberg. Some of the topics covered are:

   • the types of hospitals and how they differ
   • the "cast of characters" in the hospital, including doctors, nurses, therapists, technicians, orderlies, and so forth — and what each does
   • how to prevent infections, medical errors, and adverse drug events
   • patients' rights
   • how doctors' orders work
   • tips for faster healing

2. *How to Survive Your Hospital Stay: The Complete Guide to Getting the Care You Need — and Avoiding Problems You Don't* by Gail Van Kanegan and Michael Boyette. It lists eight ways to prepare for a hospital stay. One of these is especially worth highlighting: ensuring that you have a health care advocate, someone who can watch out for you when you can't watch out for yourself. (Or, as an article in the *Wall Street Journal* advised: "Don't go to the hospital alone, if you can possibly avoid it."[395])

It then identifies ten risks and how to avoid them. These include some not highlighted elsewhere, such as bed sores, malnutrition, surgical complications, and falls (very common for hospital patients). It also addresses another danger point, the transition from the hospital to home.

3. *Protect Yourself in the Hospital: Insider Tips for Avoiding Hospital Mistakes for Yourself or Someone You Love* by Thomas A. Sharon. This book discusses topics such as hospital ratings; what happens in emergency rooms, operating rooms, and recovery rooms; communicating effectively with the staff; and avoiding medical errors, infections, drug mistakes, and other unwanted consequences of care.

Separately, another resource that may be available to you is MTM (Medication Therapy Management). To help address potential problems with polypharmacy, services are starting to appear that will analyze your drug regimen to identify drug interactions and side effects, and provide advice. Medicare will pay for these services for some people over the age of 65 who have multiple chronic diseases, take a number of drugs, and have high drug costs.[396]

Additionally, people can purchase services to do the same thing on their own. On the web, search for medication therapy management services. It will be necessary to apply some judgment to figure out if the available offerings are reputable and worth pursuing.

Danger Spots: Post-Treatment Management

After any significant treatment, it's critical to pay attention to make sure that recovery isn't derailed. When people come home from the hospital, suddenly they're on their own. The professionals aren't there.

It is often unclear what prescriptions are duplicates; which drugs that the individual was taking before going into the hospital should be continued and which ones discontinued; what the patient is physically capable of and what can lead to injury; what the next steps are for continued care; and what else the patient needs to know to avoid big problems following a hospital stay.

One study showed that "the majority of U.S. hospitals operate the equivalent of revolving doors for their patients. One of every four heart failure patients and slightly less than one in five heart attack and pneumonia patients land back in the hospital within 30 days."[397]

The study explains: "Rehospitalization is a frequent, costly, and sometimes life-threatening event that is associated with gaps in follow-up care."[398] That means, for instance, that once discharged from the hospital, the patients did not see their doctors to make sure that they knew what to do next given whatever happened in the hospital.

One reason that this transition hasn't received more attention? "Getting hospitals to be more efficient about ensuring that patients see their doctors after surgery may be difficult, as returning patients represent returning business."[399] Said another way, hospitals earn more if patients are readmitted.

Two booklets are available for download from www.caregiving.org/pubs/brochures.htm:

- "Hospital Discharge Planning: Helping Family Caregivers Through the Process"
- "A Family Caregiver's Guide to Hospital Discharge Planning"

Cost and Quality Websites

The federal government hosts:

- Hospital Compare, at www.hospitalcompare.hhs.gov/ to report on the quality of care in U.S. hospitals and the costs of having a procedure done at one hospital compared to another
- Nursing Home Compare, at www.medicare.gov/nhcompare/ to report on the quality of nursing homes

The Joint Commission offers comprehensive quality reports about virtually all health care organizations in the U.S. through its Quality Check program, available at http://www.jointcommission.org. The Joint Commission is a national organization that sets standards and evaluates the performance of hospitals and other care organizations. (It also plays a role overseas.)

HealthGrades at www.HealthGrades.com provides ratings of doctors, hospitals and nursing homes. While some information is available at no charge, more details are provided for a fee.

NCQA provides ratings of health insurance plans, as well as ratings of hospitals and doctors, at http://www.ncqa.org/tabid/60/Default.aspx.

Your health insurer may provide information as well.

Checklists

Many of the books and websites already mentioned offer checklists. The Joint Commission, for example, provides a great set of checklists in a series called "Speak Up" at http://www.jointcommission.org/GeneralPublic/Speak+Up/. They address topics such as how to work with your doctors to avoid medical errors; avoiding mistakes with medical tests, drugs, and surgery; and preventing infections. Other topics covered are pain management and follow-up care.

AHRQ, the federal Agency for Healthcare Research and Quality, also offers very comprehensive checklists available at http://www.ahrq.gov/consumer/safety.html.

Two of the titles offered are:

- "20 Tips to Help Prevent Medical Errors"
- "20 Tips to Help Prevent Medical Errors in Children"

Other titles give advice about preparing for medical appointments, reducing infections, and taking medicine safely.

This site also offers podcasts and videos with similar information.

The Partnership for Healthcare Excellence offers checklists it calls Fact Sheets at http://www.partnershipforhealthcare.org/resources/factsheets.asp. This site also offers an e-mail alert feature so that you can be notified when new Fact Sheets are added. Two of the titles in this series are:

- "What You Can Do to Choose the Right Doctor for You"
- "What You Can Do to Prepare for Your Doctor's Appointment"

Other titles offer advice on preparing for surgery, taking medicine safely, staying healthy, and preventing infection.

The site also offers a "One Stop Guide to Quality Health Care" which provides links to dozens of other sites that can help you address topics such as choosing a doctor, comparing hospitals, arranging advance directives/hospice care, and understanding health care quality in general.

For instance, one of the links under general health care quality is "Navigating the Health Care System," which is an Agency for Healthcare Research and Quality offering which includes articles such as "How to Complain — And Get Heard."

Your insurer may also offer checklists and other resources.

Decision Aids

When you are faced with a potentially life-threatening condition, it may be hard to know what questions to ask or how to organize your thoughts. Decision aids can help. They highlight key questions to ask or issues to consider. Some decision aids compare treatment options for a particular condition in plain language, identifying the benefits and risks of each.

The idea of providing decision aids to patients is not as widespread as would be ideal. Here are two examples of websites that do provide such aids:

- http://decisionaid.ohri.ca/decguide.html provides both a generic decision aid and a decision aid specific to each of about 100 different medical conditions. The site is unusual in that for each decision aid, it provides answers to 30 questions about the validity of the information given. For example, it tells you whether people actually facing the decision tested the decision aid to see if it was helpful to them.
- http://www.guidesmith.org/questions-for-your-doctor/. While designed to help women with decisions about breast cancer, the questions/suggestions it offers can be readily applied to other situations. It provides an extremely comprehensive list of nearly a hundred questions/topics ranging from "decisions that need to be made now" vs. "decisions that need to be made later" to what your "hopes, fears, [and] unspoken thoughts or feelings" are.

The parent site (http://www.guidesmith.org) also provides "Seven Steps to Survive" and "Top Ten Lessons," both of which offer thoughtful insight into dealing with serious illnesses.

Fatal Assumptions

Assumptions that can get you into trouble include:

- *If they graduated from medical school, they must be good.*
  Think about your own high school or college class. Would you say that all of your classmates had equal skills and abilities? It's unlikely. There's a wide range of performance in all jobs — from the check-out clerks in your local grocery store to your child's teachers to doctors and lawyers.
- *All doctors and hospitals deliver about the same quality of care.*
  Like individual athletes or football or baseball teams, some are better than others.
- *If it costs a lot, it must be high quality.*
  If you believe that, then marketers have done their job very well. However, studies repeatedly show that cost and quality in health care are not linked.[400] Some of the most outstanding hospitals cost far less than those that provide average or poor care.

- *The newer the test or treatment, the better it is.*
  New technology used in diagnostic testing may not provide better diagnoses, and it can have higher risks. For example, building on the discussion in Chapter Ten, "CT scans [for heart disease] . . . have never been proved in large medical studies to be better than older or cheaper tests. And they expose patients to large doses of radiation, equivalent to at least several hundred x-rays, creating a small but real cancer risk."[401] Additionally, studies repeatedly show that some older cheaper drugs work better and have fewer side effects than some newer more expensive drugs.[402]
- *A doctor who orders more tests and treatments is better than one who does less.*
  As suggested by the discussion in Chapter Two, this is a dangerous assumption. "As much as half of the $2.3 trillion spent today [on health care in the U.S.] does nothing to improve health," is how the CEO of one health care organization puts it.[403]
- *There's no harm in having a test done.*
  Tests can cause harm all by themselves; they can also lead to more tests and unnecessary treatments, some of which may cause harm as well. If there is no good reason to have a test, it might be good to think twice before agreeing to it.
- *It's always better to see a doctor instead of a nurse.*
  That's a view not supported by the data. For example, "Patient health outcomes were similar for nurses and doctors but patient satisfaction was higher with nurse-led care. Nurses tended to provide longer consultations [and] give more information to patients."[404] Similarly, "Patients were more satisfied with care by a nurse practitioner [compared to care by a doctor]. . . . No differences in health status were found."[405]

In general, when considering assumptions like the above, it would be good to ask: What's the evidence to support that view?

CHAPTER SIXTEEN

Chaos

The U.S. health care system is on the verge of collapsing under its own weight. This unstable environment creates openings for enterprising people and organizations to offer new approaches to dealing with old problems. Some of these are brilliant innovations. Others are ineffective or destructive. If the three changes described in Chapter Fourteen are slow in coming, expect to see even more new efforts surface in an attempt to address the health care crisis — or to profit from the chaos.

Unintended Consequences of Mandates

People responsible for a pot of money often put controls in place to try to stop other people from spending too much of it. That's understandable. However, the approaches they use sometimes cause other problems.

For instance, in a classic case, a number of years ago the state of New Hampshire limited Medicaid patients to a maximum of three prescriptions drugs at any time.[406] Their logic was clear: drug costs had been rising at an alarming rate and they needed to contain them.

They succeeded in cutting drug costs. However, the use of emergency services and hospitalization increased — and the cost *increases* that resulted were 17 times greater than the cost *decreases* from the reduced use of drugs.[407]

In 2009, proposed health care legislation would cut payments to doctors if they provided more tests and treatments to their patients than did 90% of other physicians with patients like theirs.[408] It's clear that way too many tests and treatments are ordered. It's clear that something needs to be done to get that pattern to stop.

However, as one doctor noted, the kind of restriction being proposed is a "blunt instrument." A possible outcome is that doctors refuse to treat really sick patients, believing that they will end up taking a pay cut if they do so.[409]

That is, doctors won't really change their approach to treatment; they'll simply select patients whose treatment, they believe, will keep them off the "trouble" list. It's not clear that this solution is especially useful.

Getting Ahead of the Science

A time-honored tool used to change behavior is taxes. For instance, research shows that every 10% increase in taxes on cigarettes yields a drop of 4% in smoking across the board — and about an 8% drop in smoking in adolescents.[410] In New York State, the tobacco tax was raised by $1.25 per pack in 2008. A year later, the percentage of adults who smoked was reported as 16.7%, a drop of 12%.[411]

Policy makers are thinking about applying this concept more broadly. One proposal calls for "imposing a tax on sugar sweetened beverages . . . [such as] soft drinks, iced tea and iced coffee, sports drinks and fruit drinks."[412]

A possible result is that people will switch to artificially sweetened drinks. It's not clear that this change will improve their health. In an article titled, "Artificial Sweetener Linked to Weight Gain," the conclusion given is that "Food containing artificial sweeteners may be fattening instead of slimming, according to a study that found rats given yogurt with [an artificial sweetener] gained more weight than those eating the sugar-sweetened variety."[413]

It goes on to note that "The rise in worldwide obesity correlates with a jump in artificial sweetener use." It also reports that "Earlier research has suggested that people who drink diet soda have higher blood sugar, low levels of good cholesterol and abnormal fats."[414] Another article — reporting on different research — notes that while "a calorie is a calorie . . . certain foods seem to fuel the appetite like pouring gasoline on a fire."[415] One of these foods is artificial sweeteners.[416]

Thus, an unintended consequence of a law intended to help reduce obesity is that it may instead help increase it. Over time, it is likely that other laws will be proposed that also have unintended consequences.

Using Money to Drive Your Behavior

Your insurer or employer may use financial incentives to encourage you to do things which they believe will improve your health. The government is trying to help them.

Federal laws proposed in 2009 would allow employers to offer discounts on health insurance premiums of up to 50% to employees for meeting specific goals "such as keeping their weight, cholesterol, and blood pressure within healthy ranges."[417]

Said another way, if you don't meet the goals, you could end up paying twice as much for your health insurance as the person sitting at the next desk.[418] Just as is the case with the work you do, you may not have complete control over everything needed to meet your objectives, but you may be held accountable for the results anyway.

An article in the *New England Journal of Medicine* noted that genetics accounts for 30% of health outcomes, and social circumstances and environmental exposure account for another 20%. Your behavior drives 40%, and the health care you get drives the final 10%.[419]

Said another way, you may be able to change less than half of the equation. However, the person with the biggest impact on your health is you; realistically, you're the obvious person to hold accountable. Still, it may be hard to accept the idea that your employer sets goals for *your body* that you have to meet, or else your pay is affected. Even if the goals are ones you agree with, the fact that somebody else sets them can be unsettling.

In another example of using money to drive behavior, one insurer gives people who promptly refill certain prescriptions a $20 discount off their next prescription.[420] This move is consistent with the picture painted in Chapter Five: the presumption is that all drugs prescribed work for everyone and have no side effects. Thus, insurers and others try to come up with ways to get you to take all drugs as prescribed.

Other variations on financial incentives are likely to surface. One can imagine a plan that requires standard cancer screening tests at regular intervals. If you don't get those tests, and then end up with an advanced case of cancer, you might find yourself on the hook for treatment costs.

Or perhaps you are offered an asthma treatment plan. Participate, and your regular insurance terms apply. Decline to participate, and your share of the costs to manage your disease — and deal with any emergencies — rises dramatically.

Financial incentives all reflect two elements. The first is the desire to get you to take more responsibility for your own health (and related frustration that many people don't seem to be doing so.) The second element is the belief that the way to change that picture is to create financial rewards and penalties.

This framework invites you to make the focus of your thinking about your health largely financial, instead of having it be about enabling you to lead the life you want.

This perspective may reflect what matters to the people paying, but it doesn't necessarily reflect what matters most to you — and you're the main actor. This discrepancy means that these solutions may be appealing in the short run but are not likely to be very successful in the long run — at least if the goal is for you to take genuine responsibility for your own health.

Money

Extrinsic (external) rewards such as money can change people's behavior when the task being rewarded is very simple and requires little original thinking.[421] (As an analogy, a rat hitting a lever to dispense food pellets comes to mind.)

However, two pitfalls are worth noting. First, when a task requires more complex thinking, creativity, or engagement from the individual, extrinsic rewards actually result in *worse* performance.[422]

Second, once people are used to getting paid to do something, their interest in the task drops and their intrinsic (internal) motivation to do it *decreases*.[423] Paying children to read, for example, has typically been found to reduce their interest in reading. Some high-paid athletes have a similar experience regarding their passion for their sport.[424]

In many cases, "rewards to encourage participation in an activity, solving a problem, or completing a task . . . are . . . found to decrease self-determination. This decline in autonomy, along with the perception that the motivator is controlling, account for extensive decreases in intrinsic motivation. (Akin-Little, Eckert, Lovett, & Little, 2004)."[425]

Other researchers echo this conclusion.

"External rewards for performing an activity or meeting a standard are viewed as controlling, according to intrinsically [internally] motivated people. This external motivation approach is perceived as more of a restraint on self-determination, or independence, than a reward for achieving the goal. Achievement-based rewards can also pressure an individual to perform up to an expected standard. All of these feelings contribute to a decrease in intrinsic motivation (Cameron, Pierce, Banko, & Gear, 2005)."[426]

In other words, being paid for participating in health-related activities or achieving health-related goals might lead you to feel even less as if you are CEO of your own health and health care. Said another way, these payments in the long run may decrease your overall interest in taking responsibility for your health because it feels like someone else is calling the shots and imposing on you their ideas about what matters.

That said, the use of such rewards will continue and even expand because they help the people who are paying for health care both to change your behavior and to cut their costs — in the short run.

To Pay or Not To Pay

People who pay for health care are making a variety of attempts to pay for care that works and to not pay for care that doesn't work. For instance, Medicare will no longer pay hospitals for treating some bed sores, some blood clots and infections resulting from hospital care, consequences of leaving unintended foreign objects inside a patient during surgery, patient falls, and a host of other "never events."[427] They are termed "never events" because they are never supposed to happen.

On a related but different note, in a bid to have their drugs covered by insurers, some pharmaceutical companies are changing how they charge for their drugs, so that insurers pay only when patients using a particular drug actually improve with treatment.[428]

In the short run, one can guess that these agreements will lead to even more efforts to get people to take their drugs as prescribed. That move could create problems for many people. They may be pressured to take drugs which don't work for them or which cause serious side effects, as discussed in Chapter Five.

In the longer run, though, agreements like this are likely to lead to some improvements in drug prescribing practices. More of an effort will probably be made to find ways to tell up front if specific individuals are likely to be helped or hurt by a particular treatment. If there's no way to tell up front, then there will be a focus on monitoring people carefully to see how they are doing on the drug.

Carrying the concept of holding doctors and hospitals accountable for what happens when they treat people, one can picture payments in the future varying depending on how good the hospital or doctor is.

For example, if one hospital has an infection rate of 6% and one has an infection rate of 1%, the one with the lower rate might command higher prices. At the same time, your health insurer might set a co-pay for you for using the hospital with lower infection rates at perhaps $100, while your co-pay if you choose to go to the other hospital might be $500. That is, they might encourage you to get better care by making it cost you less.

The same type of payment differences might be applied to doctors. If you choose to go to a doctor known to get better results, you might have a smaller co-pay.

New Models of Care

New options for care that you may run across include retail clinics, medical tourism, telemedicine, group visits (Shared Medical Appointments), concierge (or boutique) medicine, and e-mail consultations. Each of these is described below.

Retail Clinics

Retail clinics are the 7-Elevens of health care: they have convenient locations and hours; they are easy to deal with; they intentionally limit what they sell. The analogy breaks down in a couple of ways: first, the prices in retail clinics are *lower* than the prices at the full-service alternative (your doctor's office.)[429] Second, retail clinics are way out ahead of traditional doctors' offices in record-keeping.[430]

Retail clinics are deliberately designed to be patient-centric. For example, they are located inside big stores that you are likely to visit anyway, such as Wal-Mart and Walgreens. Many of them even provide beepers so that you can shop until it's your turn to be seen.[431]

Other characteristics of the 1000+ retail clinics operating today:

- No appointment is needed. Wait times are relatively short.
- Typical staff are NPs (nurse practitioners), who have more training than nurses but less than doctors.
- Treatment follows nationally recognized standards for optimal care for any given condition, and conditions treated are a subset of what a doctor would treat.
- Records are kept electronically, which means two things: first, the clinics have a way to track diagnoses and treatment, so they can *ensure* that they are providing the nationally recognized treatment for any given diagnoses; second, each patient walks out with a printout summarizing the day's visit.
- They actively encourage people to establish a relationship with a primary care doctor.
- Retail clinics tend to equal or out-perform all other sites of care — including doctors' offices and emergency rooms — on every measure, according to a recent independent research study.[432]

Retail clinics sometimes elicit opposition from doctors. Many dire predictions have been made about the dangers to patients of using these facilities. None of these predictions has been proven true.[433] In fact, as the study referenced above revealed, quality of care is the same or *better* in a retail clinic than in the typical traditional doctor's office.

Retail clinics are viewed by some doctors as unfair competition. If health care were individual-centric — if its focus were on enabling you to lead the life you want — then this argument would be off the table. Providing people with an inexpensive high quality way to get basic routine care — when they are unable to see their primary care doctor — would be viewed as an entirely constructive option.

Long Distance Care

Time and geography are falling as barriers to care, at least in some cases:

- *Medical tourism* involves traveling a significant distance from home for elective care such as joint replacement.[434] Care may be provided in distant locales such as Thailand or India, often by U.S.-trained doctors in hospitals accredited by the same U.S.-based organization that accredits U.S. hospitals. Quality can be excellent and costs may be 15%-85% lower than for the same procedure done in the U.S.[435] About 750,000 Americans went abroad for care in 2007.[436]
- *Telemedicine* typically involves either the doctor/nurse and patient in one location, consulting a doctor at another location via high-definition video,[437] or doctors/nurses contacting — via telephone or the internet — patients who are homebound or who live far from medical care.[438]

Both of these innovations can help you get better care at a price you can afford. As with any service that you might buy, it's important to be a thoughtful shopper to increase the odds that the care you buy will meet your needs.

Attention

Two innovations in how care is provided may also be useful. On the face of it, they appear to be opposites. The first is group visits (also known as Shared Medical Appointments), in which perhaps a dozen patients meet with the doctor simultaneously. The second is concierge (or boutique) medicine, in which the doctor limits the number of patients he takes, and charges a flat annual fee to be available 24/7 to provide or coordinate any needed care.

Group appointments, at first glance, sound ridiculous: you and a dozen or so other patients with the same condition — diabetes, for example — meet with the doctor at the same time? How is that supposed to work? But it can work spectacularly well, even better than traditional one-on-one visits, for two reasons.

The first is that because the appointments are typically for ninety minutes, a great deal of ground can be covered and many questions can be answered that normally the doctor doesn't have time to address. The second is that patients can and do learn from each other. Recall from Chapter Twelve the absence of any insight for Shannon into how other people with MS coped with their condition. Having a chance to hear about other people's experiences can be a huge win.

One approach, called Drop-In Group Medical Appointments, or DIGMA, involves a standing appointment once a week for people with a particular condition. Patients with that condition are welcome to come, but they aren't obliged to. Typically, they show up if they have a question or need something specific.[439]

Because they can count on getting care at a certain time each week, it's less nerve-wracking for them. They don't face delays in getting appointments.

Group medical appointments, to be done right, require a huge amount of organization on the part of the doctor's office. Professionals in the room for the appointment — which takes place in a large meeting room — include one or more nurses to take vital signs and perform other hands-on checks; a "documenter" who captures all the necessary information for each patient's chart; the doctor; and others as appropriate. For example, one of these might be a specialist in behavior change who can help people figure out how to get necessary changes to work in their lives. Another might be a dietician.

Interestingly, one study shows that patient satisfaction is much higher for people who attend group appointments. Seventy-four percent rated their care "excellent." People who saw the very same doctors one-on-one rated their care "excellent" only 59% of the time.

Further, 87% of those who participated in one group appointment said that they wanted their next visit to be a group appointment as well.[440]

Seemingly at the other end of the spectrum is concierge medicine. In this model, doctors typically charge a flat fee ranging from $1,500/year to $10,000/year or more[441] to provide preventive and routine care with much more time and attention than are common today. Services include lengthier office visits (30 minutes is typical), same-day appointments, 24/7 access to the doctor, intensive care coordination if you need to see specialists or are in the hospital, and other services intended both to increase your peace of mind and to help you get better outcomes.

If concierge medicine interests you and you find a doctor in your area who offers it, one critical question to ask is what exactly is covered by the flat fee you pay. Generally, fees at the higher end of the scale cover *all* the costs of any primary care needed; the doctor does not accept insurance. You would still need insurance or other funds to cover hospital care, drugs, and specialists.[442]

Fees at the lower end of the scale generally tend to cover: more time in office visits, greater access to the doctor, care coordination, and prevention/wellness coaching. "Exercise and nutrition counseling"[443] might be included. Under this model, insurance is still billed for every service it will cover.

Virtual Visits

Although this shift is slow in coming, more health plans are starting to pay for e-mail consultations, which have been shown to be more convenient for both doctors and patients, and more cost-effective for insurers.[444]

Model Questions

New ways for you to get health care are likely to continue to surface. Questions to ask before you embrace any of them include:

- How is this different from what I get today?
  - What about it is better than what I get today? Said another way, how does this approach do a better job of enabling me to lead the life I want?
  - What about it would critics say is worse than what I get today?
- If I don't like it, can I go back to what I had before?
- What am I giving up by going this route?
- How does the cost differ from what I pay today?

Playing Games

While some health care professionals and policy makers are trying to influence your behavior with financial rewards and penalties, others are taking a different — and probably more constructive — approach. It involves engaging people in activities that they find appealing — and that have health benefits as well. An article in *Health Affairs* explains:

"Digital games, including virtual realities, computer simulations, and online play… make health care fun." Some of these games, such as Dancetown, encourage activity such as dancing "on a digitized footpad, following a set of visual and musical cues from a computer."[445]

The wildly popular Wii Sports and Wii Fit Plus systems, with a variety of games/activities available, are other examples of offerings that integrate physical activity with appealing computer programs.

Other games are designed to educate specific patient populations — people with diabetes, cancer, or asthma, for example. Others address broader topics such as nutrition. Done well, these games are successful at engaging people, improving their self-care, decreasing emergency room visits, and improving medical outcomes — all without lecturing or giving people lengthy, unpalatable lists of do's and don'ts.[446]

Another variant that builds on people's enthusiasm for games gives children wireless pedometers. A computer program uploads the number of steps they have taken. Those steps provide the "power" to run an online game. The more they have walked, the longer they can play.[447]

One expert explains the evolution in thinking: "The first wave was, 'We've got to change people's behavior' to help them avoid chronic disease. . . . That failed because people didn't like being told what to do. . . . The second wave was, 'Let's take healthy behaviors and make them more fun.' So we added a television to a treadmill. . . . The third wave is, 'We're thinking about the things people already love to do, and we're adding health to those things. We're connecting with their lifestyles, not telling them what to do.'"[448]

This trend is a huge win, for two reasons. First, it's more effective than traditional efforts in helping people to change their behavior. Second, it indicates that an important philosophical shift is underway: designing care around the needs/learning style/preferences of the individual — rather than around the mindset of health care experts. It's the difference between *controlling* people and *engaging* them.

CHAPTER SEVENTEEN

The Future When Health Care Is About You

When health care is about you, you will be treated with respect. That's a simple statement, easy to toss off. Understood deeply, though, it will change the foundations of health care. Elements of the equation that will change include: priorities for research; assumptions about your ability to understand health care; the kinds of restrictions lawmakers and insurers create; physician education; and the roles of various players in the delivery of health care.

Research

Priorities for research will concern five areas:

- placebo responders
- behavior change
- individual risk assessment
- co-morbidities (multiple diseases in the same person)
- communication

Each of these is discussed below.

Placebo Responders

As discussed in Chapter Five, some people get better even when they are given placebos, or sugar pills, which don't have any active drug ingredients. Listen to how these people are described: "They are the people who ruin clinical trials for drug companies: placebo responders, who get better on sugar pills. Drug makers want to get rid of them [exclude them from clinical trials]."[449]

Consider that perspective: these people *ruin* health care research by getting better. What would happen if they were accorded more respect? The story of Alexander Fleming offers some hints.

Researchers have long performed experiments that involved growing organisms in the lab. They were sometimes annoyed and disheartened when their experiments were ruined by an unknown fungus which killed off the organisms they were trying to grow. In exasperation, they would toss the ruined experiments into the trash.

In 1928 Alexander Fleming, a researcher more thoughtful than most, thought to ask what the mold was that killed one of his cultures — and thus discovered penicillin.[450] (It took until 1945 to develop an effective version that could be manufactured on a large scale.)[451]

In the future when health care is about you, placebo responders will be revered rather than reviled. Instead of being metaphorically tossed in the trash for ruining the experiment, they will be studied. The goal will be to discover how this great miracle occurs: they get better without heavy-duty drugs or surgery, and so avoid the potential dangers of treatment — side effects and complications — as well as the cost and inconvenience.

Researchers would work to see if anything could be learned from the way placebo responders heal in order to help others do the same. Since it's not clear that the answers would lead to sales of drugs or medical devices, such research would need to be funded and/or run by non-business organizations, such as the National Institutes of Health.

Outside of drug trials, other glimpses of the placebo response are fascinating as well, for the potential they suggest to improve health. In one study, a number of hotel housekeepers were told that their daily work — changing bed sheets and cleaning bathrooms — was a healthy workout.

In the four weeks after hearing that message, they lost an average of two pounds and saw modest improvements in their blood pressure, body fat, and BMI (Body Mass Index, a common measure of fitness). Housekeepers in the control group weren't told anything about their work and their fitness. Their weight, blood pressure, and other fitness measures were unchanged after four weeks.[452]

In the case of some surgical procedures, sham surgery — where the patient is prepped for surgery and incisions are made but the actual surgical repairs are not done — gets results that are equal to those of the real surgery.[453]

While this fact is often used to argue that the real surgery involved in the study is ineffective and shouldn't be paid for, it appears that little research has gone into exploring what exactly it is that accounts for the improvement experienced by the surgical placebo responders.

If health care were individual-centric, this topic would be a major research priority. It could result in great benefits to you at a fraction of the risk and cost which you face today for treatment.

Behavior Change

A second priority for research — and this one is truly huge — concerns what it takes for people to make changes in their behavior and stick with them over the long term; and what doctors, nurses, and other health care professionals can do to encourage such changes. One small piece of that equation involves finding vivid ways to talk with people about their health so that they genuinely understand what is happening. An example follows.

Age Progression

People who prepare information for CEOs know that it's critical to provide a clear picture of the issues so that CEOs can make informed decisions, even though they aren't the experts in every single topic. It is — or should be — the job of the health care system to make it very clear to people what the consequences are of following different courses of action.

Research shows that how information is presented has a big impact on whether people act on it or not. For instance, smokers who were told their lung age stopped smoking at twice the rate of those who were simply told their results on a breathing test.[454]

A lifelong smoker might be told, "You're 48, but you have the lungs of a 62-year-old. Your lung age is 62." Interestingly, even if people were told that their lung age was the same as their chronological age, they stopped smoking at twice the rate of the people who weren't told their lung age.[455]

Building on that picture, it's possible to imagine a computer model that does the equivalent of time-lapse photography *into the future* regarding health conditions and behaviors.

Individuals would start by identifying activities which they care most about being able to do. These might include working, driving, taking care of their finances, traveling, and so forth. Perhaps people select items from an extensive drop down menu.

Then three other kinds of information are added:

- their current health status, including any chronic conditions such as diabetes
- treatment options available to them
- behaviors they engage in related to diet, exercise, alcohol, tobacco, and so forth

Individuals could select different treatments and behaviors ("I eat salads every day," or "I live on cheeseburgers and fries," for example).

Then the computer model would fast-forward 10 or 20 years and calculate the odds that *they'll still be able to do each of those things that they care about.* For example, the model might report: "The probability that you will still be able to drive is 67 percent." And so forth. People could change their choices of treatments and behaviors and see how the odds change.

Providing people with these projections would be one way to help them understand the significance — in terms that matter to them — of any health issues they have, and the consequences of their choices.

Individual Risk Assessment

A third priority for research concerns how to identify which health risks have a high probability of interfering with an individual's ability to lead the life she wants, regardless of whether these are considered standard medical issues or not.

For instance: "For a 75-year-old with high blood pressure, the risk of death or serious disability resulting from a fall is just as high as the risk of death or serious disability caused by a stroke."[456]

Research shows that it's possible to tell who is at risk for falls, and steps can be taken to prevent them. However, this effort is often overlooked in caring for the elderly because falls "don't fit into the disease/specialist model of health care, which tends to focus on things like heart attacks and strokes."[457]

An example of another risk factor is malnutrition, common among the elderly — especially if they cannot drive, have difficulty getting groceries, find preparing meals to be a challenge, forget to eat, and/or face any other obstacles that prevent them from eating nutritious meals.

Research could provide insight into the most effective ways to assess individuals' real health risks and go on to provide insight about how to nip in the bud the most serious ones — even if they do not fit the traditional medical view.

Co-Morbidities (Multiple Diseases in the Same Person)

A fourth and very big priority for research concerns how to treat people who have multiple chronic conditions. "Two-thirds of people over age 65, and almost three-quarters of people over 80, have multiple chronic health conditions, and 68 percent of Medicare spending goes to people who have five or more chronic diseases . . . [but the] medical system [is] geared toward individual organs and diseases."[458]

Today these people — who most desperately need the most help — "are largely overlooked both in medical research and in the nation's clinics and hospitals. The default position is to treat complicated patients as collections of malfunctioning body parts rather than as whole human beings. . . . And treating one disease in isolation . . . can make another disease worse."[459]

Research in this area would need to be funded by non-business organizations — probably again the National Institutes of Health or other government-funded entity, for two reasons. First, the focus isn't on a particular drug or medical device. Second, through Medicare the government is paying most of the bills that result from not having good answers for treating people with multiple diseases, so the federal government has the biggest incentive to address the situation.

Communication

A fifth priority for research concerns how to communicate with people to accomplish two goals. The first goal is to identify and reduce the "risk and uncertainty" that the health care system traditionally transfers to the patient[460] in each of the fourteen steps in the process of health care discussed in Chapter Twelve.

An example of the kind of change that might spring from that research involves keeping people informed about wait times in an ER: "Patients who waited more than four hours to see a doctor, but felt well-informed about the delay, scored more than twice as high on overall satisfaction as those who waited just an hour but considered communication to be 'very poor.'"[461]

In other words, *knowing* what is happening dramatically improves people's experience in dealing with health care, even if the *facts* about what is happening aren't ideal.

Another example of research that would be useful concerning communicating with people to reduce their uncertainty is to figure out what they most need to know about how the hospital works when they are admitted.

For instance, if you are lying in your room and hit the call button, how long should you expect to wait for your call to be acknowledged? A minute? Twenty minutes? How long should it take for someone to come to your aid? Five minutes? An hour? What can you do if you feel you need help faster? And so forth.

The second goal for research into communication is to figure out how to communicate in ways that are likely to engage and energize people — as opposed to discouraging and deflating them. Some of the fixes likely to surface require, primarily, a change in attitude. They do not require a lot of money or high tech equipment.

As an example, contrast the response of the doctor told that fluid had continued coming out of my ear with the response of a doctor when I asked whether a mineral supplement might be interfering with the action of a particular drug. In both cases, the situation described was something that they had never seen before. (Granted, the two situations were very different in terms of how surprising they were.)

First response, instantaneous and emphatic: "That's ridiculous! That didn't happen!"

Second response, after a thoughtful pause of a few seconds: "I've never run across that. But anything is possible. I learn new things from my patients every day."[462] The second response is far more likely to engage and encourage the individual than is the first response.

The second response, by the way, comes from a doctor at the Mayo Clinic, where they have honed to a fine point the art and science of treating patients with respect. They don't do everything perfectly all the time; they just do a dramatically better job than the vast majority of other health care organizations with which I am familiar.[463]

Assumptions about Your Ability to Engage: Sy Syms and John Madden

Sy Syms was the chairman of Syms, a chain of clothing stores that sell designer and other brand clothing at discount prices. Their television ads long featured Sy Syms declaring, "An educated consumer is our best customer!" He meant that if people understood the labels Syms sells and how low his prices were compared to those in department stores, they would buy a lot of clothing from his stores.

Sometimes it seems as if the health care system is the anti-Sy Syms of your life: "An *uneducated* consumer is our best customer!" In other words, the less you know, the easier it is for doctors to perform a high volume of tests and treatments. (One patient started to ask questions about an operation her cardiologist was scheduling for her. He had said nothing about the risks or benefits of the surgery. His reply? "Honey, all you need to worry about is if I am going to listen to opera or Steely Dan during the procedure.")[464]

Contrast that picture with John Madden's approach to talking with fans about football. Upon the retirement of the legendary football broadcaster, he was hailed by the *Wall Street Journal* as "a transformational figure. . . . Mr. Madden gave the average fan credit for wanting to know more than just who caught the ball. . . . Mr. Madden was a fount of deep and complex instruction, using state-of-the-art computer graphics, scribbling circles and arrows into a freeze frame, to illustrate his lengthy explanations."[465]

The article continued: "This kind of analysis had been thought too complicated for the average fan, but Mr. Madden showed that fans not only tolerated that level of depth, but actively wanted it. His example quickly spread across [other] televised sports. . . . Mr. Madden raised the intelligence level of sports announcing. . . . John Madden's retirement should remind us that we can do better."[466]

It's possible to make people smarter about clothing and football by offering them intelligent, informed insight into what they're seeing. Why is it assumed that the same is not true about people's health and health care? If health care treated people with more respect — gave them a little more credit — it would take for granted that they are:

- able to be a critical source of essential information about themselves and their health
- capable of absorbing important information
- able to make good choices

The following two sections suggest changes consistent with this thinking. These could occur in a future in which health care is about you.

Risk and Uncertainty

Two facets of health care that are greatly misunderstood are risk and uncertainty. These would be terrific topics to address in efforts to educate and engage people more in their own care.

Many people seem to believe that medical treatments are, or can be, free of risk. This belief does not line up with the facts. It's possible to die even as a result of drinking too much water.[467] There is no free lunch in medical interventions: every treatment has risks.

Some people feel betrayed when the treatment they get creates problems such as pain or immobility. They had believed that a good outcome was essentially guaranteed. Their outrage has at its root the fact that doctors tend to focus on the "treatment works, no side effects" possibility, which is only one of *four* likely outcomes when people are treated. (See the chart in Chapter Five.)

On the other end of the spectrum, some people avoid *all* medical tests and treatments because they recognize, quite accurately, that they have risks.

People who ignore risks may pursue too much medical care because the only part of the picture they see is the list of potential benefits. People who focus *only* on the risks may avoid needed treatment because they don't seriously consider how it may help them. Neither of these approaches to risk is likely to lead to the best outcomes.

Education about risk would include a discussion of *comparative* risks. For example, when I had the brain fluid leak, there were serious risks associated with the surgery — but without the surgery, I was almost certain to die. Thus, having the surgery was the *less risky* choice.

People also are generally unaware of the uncertainties in medicine. It would be very helpful for them to understand the highlights about what is *known* and what is *not known* about their condition and about proposed tests or treatments. For example, is it *known* whether a treatment they're considering keeps people alive longer? Or is that an unknown? That knowledge can help them make thoughtful choices.

General education about risk and uncertainty in health care might be provided through insurers, employers, and federal and state health care programs (Medicare and Medicaid). Integrated health care systems (which provide care ranging from primary care doctors' visits to hospitalization) might also provide this education for the people they serve.

Drug Labels

A second initiative that assumes that people can understand clear information involves using a standard format to present facts about drugs: "What if consumers could calculate the benefits and risks of taking a prescription drug as easily as they can gauge the carbs and calories of an Oreo cookie? Inspired by the nutrition fact panels on food packaging, researchers . . . [propose] a similar concept — numerical tables that quantify the benefits of taking a drug compared with a placebo, and that list the odds of having side effects."[468]

This approach would be a great step forward.

Better Treatment, Lower Cost — Without Treatment Restrictions

It's common to hear stories about seemingly arbitrary limits that health insurers place on what treatments they will pay for. If rules are necessary, what is a more respectful alternative to mandating treatment limits? Mandating *that patients be included* in the decision-making process that determines what is going to be done to them. This is a third way in which assuming that people can be educated about their health and health care can yield better results.

As noted in Chapter Five, one study concluded that people had any say at all in their treatment only 9% of the time.[469] When they are given meaningful information about different treatment options — and the opportunity to choose — "they tend to choose less-invasive and less-expensive treatments than they would have otherwise received."[470]

Research shows that doctors often don't describe risks of testing or treatments.[471] The new mandate would require that people be presented with both *risks* and *benefits* of each proposed test or treatment and, where appropriate, the risks and benefits of other possible testing and treatment options, including the option of having no test or treatment. To make the inclusion of patients work, it is necessary that the information presented:

- Be unbiased.
- Be written in language that most people can understand. That requirement generally means that it should be written at a fourth grade reading level.[472] It is entirely possible to convey complex health information at a fourth grade level.
- Be laid out in a way that makes it easy to compare the options. E.g., a chart might show key facts about each choice: benefits, risks, how success is defined, success rates, and unknowns.

- Describe outcomes in terms relevant to the average reader. That is, not "will have debrided the patellar tendon" but instead "will be able to walk around the block without pain."

Decision Quality

Doctors sometimes worry that patients will make really bad decisions if given the chance.[473] Yes, they might. If they do, it may mean that the risks and benefits of the different options haven't been explained clearly enough to them.

Another possibility is that they have priorities and concerns that lead them to draw a conclusion different from the one doctors draw. Typically, no one asks them. If they were regarded with more respect, they would be asked.

Drug Feedback Loops

Related to the idea of mandating that *patients be included* in making treatment choices is the idea of mandating a *feedback loop* when certain drugs are prescribed, rather than mandating or denying *specific drugs*.[474] The purpose of the feedback loop is to see whether drugs prescribed for chronic diseases are helping the patient without causing serious side effects.

Some thought could be given to defining consistent minimum standards that this feedback loop would need to meet.[475] (See the discussion of feedback loops in Chapter Twelve.)

Physician Education

What medical education today generally *produces* is doctors who:

- specialize in specific fields like heart disease or joint problems
- are trained by treating people primarily in hospitals
- expect to call the shots

What the health care system *needs* is more doctors who:

- focus on caring for the whole patient
- emphasize prevention
- support people (who are CEOs of their own health and health care) in making behavior changes and treatment choices that will increase the odds that they can lead the lives they want

Either the way in which doctors are created needs to change, or doctors need to accept a lesser role in health care, and other health care professionals need to be created who can oversee patient care in a way that will address the above critical needs.

If doctors want to continue to play a leading role, then three aspects of medical training will change: content of the class work, content of hands-on training, and the selection of students (future doctors).

First, a revamp of the classroom curriculum is needed to reflect your legitimate health care needs.[476] Topics added or receiving more emphasis will include:

- the purpose of health care: *to enable people to lead the lives they want*
- what drives health: that is, 40% is behavior, 30% is genetics, and so forth
- the incidence and prevalence of unintended consequences in health care — for example, the percentage of all deaths caused by health care
- patient population characteristics such as the percentage of people admitted to hospitals who are over age 65; the percentage of people with multiple medical problems; and the percentage of deaths due to chronic disease
- what individual-centric health care looks like: individuals are CEOs of their own health and health care and the health care system plays a supporting role
- what respect and disrespect in interactions with patients look like and how these affect the outcomes of care
- situational leadership: the idea that one size does not fit all; some people will want to take on more responsibility for decisions than others will, and some will want to take on less — the doctor needs to be flexible
- process management: for example, the need to connect the dots in order to get the intended results
- care coordination: why it is needed; doctors' role
- roles in health care delivery: patient, doctor, nurse, nurse practitioner, physician assistant, social worker, pharmacist, physical therapist, dietician, health coach, chiropractor, patient advocate, and so forth, and what each of these is expected to do
- prevention and management of chronic conditions
- psychology of patient behavior and how to help people make behavior changes
- special requirements for the care of the many people with multiple health issues: deciding the priorities for treatment, recognizing the dangers of polypharmacy, and so forth[477]
- geriatrics: issues unique to the care of the elderly that require different actions and behaviors on the part of doctors;[478] the philosophy of "slow medicine"[479]

Second, a modification of hands-on training is needed to shift some training time from hospital settings to primary care, nursing homes, and hospice care.

Third, a change in admission standards is needed to produce more doctors whose perspectives and interests are a better fit with the most common medical needs people have today. Health care still needs brain surgeons — I can attest to that. The issue is that the ratio of specialists to generalists is skewed today.

Roles in Care Delivery

Diagnostic efforts and roles in primary care are likely to change. Attempts to address the labor shortage in health care will require solutions other than "produce more doctors." You yourself are likely to take on a new and larger role in a way not previously mentioned. The following sections describe these changes.

Diagnostics: A New Specialty

When health care is about you, diagnostics will be a recognized field of its own. Diagnosticians will be trained to pay very careful attention to the symptoms patients describe, and will use sophisticated computer systems to aid them in coming up with accurate diagnoses.

Any individual who is not clearly achieving agreed-upon treatment goals after faithfully following an appropriate treatment regimen for a short period of time — days, weeks, or months, depending on the medical condition — will be referred to a diagnostician.

Many health care professionals would argue that only a specialist in a given field knows enough to diagnose people accurately. The problem with that argument is that it assumes that it is already known that the individuals' medical issues fall within a particular field.

When diagnoses are elusive, two of the main reasons are: first, faulty assumptions have been made about which body part is the root cause; second, the problem is not located in just one organ or body system. In both of these cases, having someone with a broader view take a fresh look at the situation can help.

Diagnosticians will work closely with individuals to train them to be keen observers of their own experience so that they can report accurately the critical information that the diagnostician needs to nail down a hard-to-diagnose condition.

On a related note, the default position when people fail to get better under their current treatment plans will *stop* being to assume that they are mentally ill, that they don't want to get better, or that they are lying. These are common views today.[480] The default position will be that medical science isn't sophisticated enough to figure out their problem yet, or hasn't come up with a solution that works for them.

Primary Care

If the focus in medical schools does not change, then primary care will cease to be the province of doctors. Nurses, nurse practitioners, physicians' assistants, and new players such as "health coaches" will be the first point of entry for most people into the health care system.[481]

A former government official who used to run the U.S. Department of Health and Human Services, commenting on the shortage of primary care doctors, noted that "there will be opportunities for nurses to take on a larger role in offering primary care."[482]

In fact, one doctor with impressive credentials, who has advised the White House on health policy, proposes going even further. In an article titled, "The Grandparents Corps: A New Primary Care Model," Dr. Arthur Garson notes that some doctors have said that "a good percentage of their patients could be taken care of by good grandparents."[483]

Grandparents often have common sense and experience with health care, and could be formally trained to help improve health literacy, to treat simple fevers, to help people stick with chronic care plans, and to perform other similar tasks that do not require four years of medical school. Dr. Garson goes on to propose that this idea be pursued to help alleviate the labor shortage in health care.[484]

When health care is more individual-centric, non-doctor professionals (and possibly lay people) will be trained to help people clarify their treatment goals — what life it is that they want health care to enable them to lead — and to help them understand how to change their behavior and select treatments to improve the odds that they can lead that life.

Labor Shortage

It is commonly observed that there are not enough doctors to take care of everybody.[485] Other solutions to this problem, not described above, will:

- shift care upstream
- increase the integration of care delivery
- encourage self-service

Each of these is discussed below.

Shifting care upstream means that if problems can be *prevented* — for example, if there are fewer people with heart disease or diabetes because people change their behavior and avoid these conditions — then the demand for intensive treatment after a lot of damage is done will decrease over time.

That decrease would reduce the demand for specialists. Then they would have the capacity to treat all the people who today are going without care.

Pulling this shift off, of course, is seen as almost impossible to do. That's because insufficient research has gone into figuring out how to help people make behavior changes that they can stick with. As noted earlier in the chapter, this topic will be a major research priority when health care is genuinely about you. Once research starts to provide better answers, the shift towards prevention will gain momentum.

A second solution to the labor shortage may be a by-product of another change that can result in better care. That change is a shift towards integrated care delivery systems. What does that mean? It means that one organization is responsible for all of your care — from flu shots to heart transplants.

This concept makes some people nervous. However, it provides huge advantages. Typically, doctors in such systems are on salary. As a result, they have no incentive to over treat you — they don't make any more money if they do.

Additionally, such organizations typically have EMR (Electronic Medical Record) systems, which means that every doctor can immediately see all the results of every test that any other doctors ordered. They can also see the notes that every other doctor took when examining you, and the conclusions they drew. Having this information available to all the doctors who see you can save you a lot of time and money, and can improve your care or even save your life.

While not typically seen as a way to address the labor shortage, integrated systems are more efficient and thus can take care of more people with the same resources consumed by doctors' offices, hospitals, other health care professionals, and other sites of care that are not part of an integrated system.

Encourage Self-Service

A third solution to the labor shortage in health care is for individuals to do for themselves many things that health care workers now do for them. A simple example is that some doctors' offices have made it possible for people to go online and schedule their own appointments.

The stereotype of individuals as incompetent, self-centered bumblers whose increased involvement will only mess everything up surfaces here too: in one case, doctors were worried that if people could schedule their own appointments, they would abuse the privilege, coming in unnecessarily and clogging up the office.[486]

That disruption didn't happen. The main change observed is that people who schedule their own appointments honor those appointments — they show up as scheduled — at a greater rate than people who do not schedule their own appointments. In other words, allowing people to schedule their own appointments helped the doctor's office run better.[487] It also saved time on the part of the office staff. It was probably easier for the patients as well — who presumably went on line at their convenience.

Tapping Your Energy

You may play a game-changing role in the delivery of health care yourself. One way is through online social networks. These include sites such as:

- Facebook, "a global social networking website. . . . Users can add friends and send them messages, and update their personal profiles to notify friends about themselves. Additionally, users can join networks organized by city, workplace, school, and region."[488]
- Twitter, a "social networking and micro-blogging service that enables it users to send . . . text-based posts of up to 140 characters displayed on the author's profile page and delivered to the author's subscribers."[489]
- YouTube, "a video sharing website on which users can upload and share videos."[490]
- Second Life, "a virtual world . . . [where 'residents' can] explore, meet other residents, socialize, participate in individual and group activities," and so forth.[491]
- PatientsLikeMe, "a social networking health site that enables its members to share treatment and symptom information in order to track and to learn from real-world outcomes."[492]

What all of these sites have in common is that they would be empty shells without the content provided by, and interaction of, the users. Health care activity can be found on all of them, from a community called Health 2.0 on Facebook to very short videos such as "Healthiest Nation — Move" and "Healthiest Nation in One Generation" on YouTube. One observer suggested 140 potential uses for Twitter in health care, including everything from disaster alerts to weight management.[493]

Researchers identified 68 health-related sites within Second Life, with activities such as "education; training programs for physicians, nurses and medical students; an increased presence of disease-specific support and discussion groups; and fundraisers that benefit medical research (with real-world dollars going into coffers)."[494]

Of particular interest among the social networking sites is PatientsLikeMe. Founder Ben Heywood explains, "What distinguishes PatientsLikeMe is that patients share specific, structured information about their medical conditions and their treatments. This allows others to find patients who are like them, and understand what happens to real people in real life who have the disease they have and who have the same treatment program."[495]

He goes on to say, "This information helps them answer two questions: 'Given my status, what is the best outcome I can expect to achieve, and how do I get there?' and 'Can I change my outcome?'"[496] An article in the *New York Times* about PatientsLikeMe is titled, "Practicing Patients," apparently referring to the fact that the patients carefully track data and often work with their doctors to change their treatments based on what they have learned on the site.

It says, "PatientsLikeMe is a tool that allows patients to manage their disease with a sophistication and precision that would have been unimaginable just a decade ago. . . . [Its] members . . . may be the vanguard of how we all will care [for] and treat our résumé of chronic diseases. They're not typical patients, in the sense of waiting for advice from a doctor. They are, rather, co-practitioners treating their conditions and guiding their care, with possibly profound implications."[497]

Social networking sites provide examples of ways in which you might actively engage in improving your health, rather than leaving most of the information, analysis, decisions, and initiative to health care professionals. (Of course, it's important to exercise good judgment — the fact that someone has posted something online doesn't guarantee that it is either accurate or useful.)

Many people put a lot of energy into dealing with their health today. However, much of their effort is thwarted by a health care system that makes it hard for them to engage. The slower that picture is to change, the faster people will turn to other avenues like social networking sites that foster, rather than obstruct, their active engagement.

Conclusion

By reading *Killer Cure*, you've educated yourself about "the other half" of the picture in health care — the part that the health care system doesn't advertise. This story isn't about good guys and bad guys. It's about broken processes and outdated attitudes.

It's important to remember that the first half of the picture does exist — doctors, nurses, hospitals and all the other players in health care often do a spectacular job of taking care of people, improving and/or saving lives as a result.

With the perspective you've gained by reading this book, you are in a much better position to understand how to get the great benefits that health care can offer, and reduce the odds of being caught by surprise by downsides you didn't know about.

I wish you all the best in your quest for health — and for health care that enables you to lead the life you want.

READERS' DISCUSSION GUIDE

A printable version of this discussion guide is available at www.killercure.net.

Readers in discussion groups are welcome to select questions to answer from the list below; there's no need to feel that you have to answer them all.

Of course, all readers should feel free to abstain from answering any questions which they are not comfortable addressing in a group discussion. Readers should also feel free to alter the details of any examples they give as necessary to protect the privacy of family and friends.

Chapter One

1. How does your own experience, or that of family and friends, support or contradict the picture painted about deaths and injuries caused by health care?

2. Do you think that medical errors, hospital-acquired infections, post-surgery blood clots, and adverse drug events are inevitable? (One might call this the "You can't make an omelet without breaking eggs" perspective.) Why or why not?

3. Shannon scarcely left Bob's side when he was hospitalized. Explaining why, she said, "He was just lying in a crib in a room. They wouldn't necessarily hear him cry. If he needed something, it's not like he could press the call button." Can you think of an example from your life in which a health care provider put himself or herself in the patient's shoes as Shannon put herself in Bob's shoes? Should they do that? Why or why not?

4. Bob lived because Shannon noticed obscure details — whether the drug in the syringe appeared clear or cloudy and the volume of the drug in the barrel of the syringe — and spoke up. How does that story compare with your expectations about the role of patients (or their parents or other advocates) when they are hospitalized?

Chapter Two

5. What do you think accounts for the fact that nearly 10 million women are tested for cancer "in an organ that they don't have"? How would doctors need to change their thinking and behavior for this situation to change? How would the women being tested need to change?

6. One critic of the tendency to prescribe drugs to large numbers of people with mild abnormalities asked, "What if you put 250 people in a room and told them they would each pay $1,000 a year for a drug they would have to take every day, that many would get diarrhea and muscle pain, and that 249 would have no benefit? . . . How many would take that?" Would you take a drug with that profile? Why or why not?

7. Doctors often complain that *insurance companies* try to *limit* tests and treatments to foster their own financial interests rather than the patient's well-being. This chapter provides data indicating that *doctors* may *order* tests and treatments to foster their own financial interests rather than the patient's well-being. With the insurance company saying one thing and the doctor saying another, how might you go about figuring out if a proposed test or treatment is in fact likely to foster your well-being or not?

Chapter Three

8. This chapter points out that the role of the individual has shifted over time. A hundred years ago individuals didn't have to do anything for big health improvements to happen. Fifty years ago they simply had to show up so that Marcus Welby, M.D. could perform his miracles. Today they need to be CEOs of their own health and health care. Do you think that most people understand that they have this job? What needs to be done to help people learn about this new role? Whose responsibility is it to educate them about it?

9. Some health care policy makers don't quite agree with the "individual as CEO" idea. They believe that patients should be "co-pilots" or "co-producers" of their health, in partnership with their doctor. What are the advantages and disadvantages to you of viewing your health as a responsibility shared with your doctor? If it's a shared responsibility, are you both equally responsible for everything? Or do you have one set of responsibilities and the doctor another set? If so, what kinds of things are each of you responsible for? How does it work if you have more than one doctor?

10. What images does the label "patient" call up for you?

Chapter Four

11. This chapter opens with a comparison between hospital ICUs and prison camps for terrorist suspects. How did you feel when you read that section? Why?

12. Do you know people who developed ICU Psychosis or were prescribed too many drugs? What impact do you think that experience had on their long-term wellbeing?

13. Have you, or family or friends, experienced situations in which you concluded that simple, inexpensive changes on the part of care providers could make a huge difference in the patient's comfort or health? What would need to happen for these changes to be made?

14. If you had a choice, how would you like to communicate with your doctor? (In person, by phone, via e-mail, through the regular mail, or some other way.) Is there a difference between how you'd prefer to communicate and what your doctor supports?

Chapter Five

15. Have you, or friends or family, had a treatment that didn't solve the health problem or that caused side effects that outweighed the benefits of the treatment? How quickly did it become evident that there were issues with the treatment? Who noticed the problem — the patient or the doctor? What could the individual (or parent, partner, or other advocate) do differently in similar situations in the future to get a better outcome faster?

16. Research shows that when people report side effects, doctors "very often dismiss their concerns." How would you deal with the situation if that happened to you?

17. Do you feel that your job as the patient is to follow doctors' orders? Why or why not? Does your answer to that question change if the orders involve *what* treatment to have (e.g., surgery vs. physical therapy for a shoulder problem) vs. *how* to execute the treatment (e.g., take one pill four times a day for ten days)? Does your answer change if you experience side effects?

Chapter Six

18. What does one health care expert mean when he says, "Healthcare systems have always transferred uncertainty and risk to the patient?" In what ways is that view consistent or inconsistent with your experience?

19. The author describes a two-month process to get a diagnosis when endometrial cancer was a possibility. Have you or a friend or family member had an experience in which it took what seemed like a long time to be diagnosed? How would your feelings be similar to or different from the author's in such a situation? What would you do differently in dealing with the doctors?

Chapter Seven

20. How do you feel about the idea of having access to all of your own medical records? Under what circumstances would you be interested in actually reading them? Have you ever needed old medical records and been unable to get them?

21. Do you make a point of finding out if your test results are normal or not? How easy is it for you to find out? How long does it typically take to get the results? How long do you think it should take?

Chapter Eight

22. Have you, or family or friends, felt that your voice simply wasn't being heard when there was a medical problem that didn't seem to fit the doctor's expectations? What would you do if you faced a situation like this in the future?

23. How would you feel if you were prescribed a drug that caused significant weight gain? What would you do?

24. Care providers in a hospital assumed that involving families would be a drain on their time. Instead, patients got better faster and nursing turnover dropped. What do you think the role of families should be when someone is hospitalized?

25. Knowing how being discounted or belittled impacts people, what can you do if you find yourself in that situation with a health care provider?

Chapter Nine

26. How would you respond if you were in the emergency room and the staff reacted to you as they did to Stephen when he was being treated for food poisoning?

27. How would you respond if you were in the hospital and realized that the doctor was about to embark on the wrong procedure?

28. This chapter includes the quotation: "Many physicians are trained 'to think of [them]selves as little gods' and resist patients who question their authority." Faced with that reality, as well as the impact of Stockholm syndrome (which tends to shut people down to avoid angering those with power over them), what can you do to deal with the power disparity you face in dealing with the health care system?

29. Should doctors and nurses pay attention to patients' feelings when dealing with their physical disorders? Is it their job to do so, or is it up to patients to control their emotions so that the professionals can get their work done? What leads you to your conclusions?

Chapter Ten

30. What are your expectations about the role doctors play in relation to you? Do you secretly want them to be gods — all-powerful and having all the answers? What are the benefits and risks of wanting doctors to be gods?

31. Have you ever been tempted to lie to a doctor? What emotions led you to consider lying as an option? (Embarrassment? Fear? Some other feeling?) If you were giving other people advice, what would you advise about lying?

32. What examples of unintended consequences can you identify in your experiences with health care?

Chapter Eleven

33. Of the possible process gaps on your side of the equation that you might experience in relation to a visit to the doctor's office, which have you experienced? (Examples include: not making effective choices about whether to seek medical care; masking or worsening symptoms through care at home; failing to explain the problem adequately; forgetting what the doctor said; not understanding what you were told; not following the instructions even though you agreed that they made sense; being unclear about how to translate the instructions into everyday life; and not understanding why it matters whether you follow the instructions or not.) How did these process gaps affect the outcome you got?

34. Have you or friends or family experienced other process gaps in health care delivery? Why do you think these arose?

35. Identify one situation in which you might use FMEA (Failure Modes and Effects Analysis) to solve a process problem.

Chapter Twelve

36. What two questions are essential to ask before starting to fix a broken process? Why do these questions matter?

37. The author concludes that the purpose of health care today is to deliver acute interventions. Based on your experience, what do *you* think the purpose of the health care system is?

38. The author goes on to propose that the purpose of health care should be *to enable people to lead the lives they want.* What do you think it should be?

39. Dr. Don Berwick is quoted as saying "I have come to believe that we — patients, families, clinicians, and the health care system as a whole — would be far better off if we professionals recalibrated our work such that we behaved with

patients and families not as hosts in the care system, but as guests in their lives."
What does he mean by that? Do you agree with him?

40. Of the fourteen steps in the process of health care listed, which one or two seem
to you to have the biggest or most troublesome gaps? (These include: wellness,
risk assessment, prevention, early intervention, triggers, triage, diagnosis, interpretation of the meaning and impact of the diagnosis, selection of treatment,
preparation for treatment, delivery of treatment, post-treatment management,
feedback loop, and integration of episode of care into life.) If it were up to you,
what would you do to close those gaps?

41. What experience can you recall in which your health, or that of family or
friends, suffered as a result of the fact that it was very difficult for the patient to
interpret the meaning and impact of a diagnosis and figure out how to move forward? If you were advising others, what would you tell them about this step?

42. How could implementing feedback loops improve health care? What can you
do in your own health care to address this gap?

Chapter Thirteen

43. Pick one of the commonly discussed approaches to addressing the health care
crisis. (These include: Universal Coverage, Single Payer, Regulation, Cost Controls, HIT, Comparative Effectiveness, Transparency, CDHP, P4P, Focused
Care, Accountable Care Organizations, and Medical Home.) If the purpose of
health care changes to be more individual-centric, are the benefits of the
approach you picked more likely or less likely to occur? Why?

Chapter Fourteen

44. Implicit in the book is the suggestion that the problem with health care isn't primarily financial; it's primarily about who has power — who gets to set the priorities and call the shots. Do you agree? Said another way, if there were
suddenly enough money to pay for health care for everybody without any limitations, would that fix the problems identified in *Killer Cure*?

45. Why does the author use the term "revolution?" Why does she compare efforts
to change how patients are viewed to efforts that freed the slaves or granted
women the right to vote?

46. The author attributes bad outcomes in health care partly to choices that professionals in the health care system make. Do you agree? Do you think that people are generally victims of circumstances, or do you believe that they can choose
to act differently?

47. What two problems, according to the author, result from ceding so much power and control to the health care system? Do you agree?

48. Why does the book start to shift its focus from how the health care system behaves to how people served by the health care system behave?

49. What does the story *The Fisherman and His Wife* have to do with health care? Do you know people who have unrealistic expectations about what health care can do for them? Do you think that any of *your* expectations about what health care can do for you might be unrealistic?

50. What examples in your own life or those of family or friends can you think of that illustrate the impact of stress on health?

51. What one or two steps can you imagine taking to reduce or manage the stress in your life?

52. How can your health care be managed as a process if care is fragmented across many doctors, hospitals, labs, etc?

Chapter Fifteen

53. What point is the author making by drawing an analogy between computer processing thirty or forty years ago and health care today?

54. If you were going to pick one step to start with, which of the CEO responsibilities seems most appealing to you? (These include: ask questions, keep a Personal Health Record, and learn how the health care system works.)

55. Can you think of an experience you or a family member or friend has had that illustrates a problem with one of the danger spots? (These include: diagnosis, treatment options, care delivery, and post-treatment management.) What resources might you draw on in the future to help prevent a similar problem?

56. Of the many resources listed, which one or two sound the most useful to you? How do you think they might help you?

Chapter Sixteen

57. What experiences have you had of financial incentives related to your health and health care? (For example, these might include reduced insurance premiums for taking certain actions, lower co-pays for some drugs and higher co-pays for others, or other adjustments to your cost of care intended to change your decisions or behavior.) In what ways have these encouraged you to take better care of yourself? In what ways have they seemed counterproductive?

58. Have you had any experience with any of the new models of care described? (These include: retail clinics, medical tourism, telemedicine, group visits,

concierge medicine, and e-mail consultations.) If so, what did you like about the experience? What did you dislike? If you haven't tried any of these, which one seems most appealing? Why?

59. What health-related games have you or family members or friends played? How did the experience affect your health or your thinking about your health and health care?

Chapter Seventeen

60. What health improvement changes have you made that you've been able to stick with for a while? What do you feel has contributed to your success?

61. One source notes that people with multiple health problems are treated "as collections of malfunctioning body parts rather than as whole human beings. . . . And treating one disease in isolation . . . can make another disease worse." In other words, treating each body part separately can make diseases involving other body parts worse. Have you, or family or friends, experienced this problem?

62. What experiences have you had of doctors, nurses, or other health care professionals saying something to you that engaged and energized you?

63. What examples can you think of in which you, or family or friends, had a voice in deciding what test or treatment to have and decided to do something different from the doctor's initial suggestion? What led to the decision? Are you (or family or friends) glad that you made that choice? If you have not had this experience, how would you go about getting a voice in the next decision you face about a major test or treatment?

64. How have you used — or how might you use — social networking sites to help improve your health?

65. What other changes do you think will happen in health care when you are treated with more respect and when its purpose becomes *to enable people to lead the lives they want?*

Conclusion

66. The book's title, *Killer Cure*, could have more than one meaning. What does it mean to you?

67. How will you change the way you deal with your health and health care, and how you talk with others about health care, as a result of reading *Killer Cure?*

ACKNOWLEDGMENTS

The cover of *Killer Cure* was designed by Louis Dalmau. My portrait is by Linda Sue Scott.

The views presented in *Killer Cure* are my own. The book would have been much harder to write without the help of many other people. The fact that they were informative or supportive in many ways does not necessarily mean that they share the views expressed; you'd have to ask them to know for sure.

The people who read drafts of the manuscript and provided feedback to help make this a more useful book for you include: Kathy Beaudoin, Amy Bewley, Pete Bewley, Jr., Cathryn Gunther, Alisa Isaac, Cathy Kushner, Helene O'Brien, and Barbara Taptich. Many of these people provided other exceptional help as well.

Others who gave invaluable assistance or support while I developed the thinking that went into the book — and wrote it — include Connie Deutsch, Chuck Fager, Pickett Guthrie, Chapin Hartford, John Hoover, Jeff Neely, Linda Powell, Marilynn Washburn, Eric Wichems, Fran Zone, and dozens of others I apologize for not listing by name.

Some of the leaders in health care improvement whose clear voices have inspired me include Don Berwick, David Eddy, Harvey Fineberg, George Halvorson, Lucian Leape, and Arnie Milstein.

Two agents of social change whose voices resonate with me — despite the fact that they died in 1772 and 1880, respectively — are John Woolman and Lucretia Mott.

My husband, Stephen Brubaker, has served as a terrific sounding board, adopting as his own the conversation topic of making health care more individual-centric. His constant willingness to discuss this subject has been an act of breathtaking generosity, renewed almost daily — year after year. He contributed the title of the book, demonstrating both his careful listening and his complex thinking. It captures three meanings:

- *Killer cure*: the cure often kills
- Kill *or* cure: the outcome of care is a coin toss
- *Killer* cure: a take-off on "killer app" (application) in the field of computer software — something that so completely changes the game that it's hard to remember what life was like before it existed — for example, e-mail is a "killer app". The "killer cure" for health care is to adopt the purpose *to enable people to lead the lives they want*. Doing so would completely change the game.

NOTES

Chapter One: It's Not the Health Care System You Think It Is

1. This calculation combines the mutually exclusive numbers of deaths reported from medical errors (200K/year), hospital-acquired infections (99K/year), adverse drug events (125K/year), and hospitalization-caused pulmonary embolisms (200K/year). "Pulmonary embolism" is the technical term for a blood clot that travels to the lungs. These four causes total 624K deaths/year. Divided by 52 weeks, the result is 12,000 deaths/week. Sources for numbers for each of the four causes of death follow:

Paul Davies, "Fatal Medical Errors Said To Be More Widespread," *Wall Street Journal*, 27 July 2004. "A new study coming out today estimates that the number of patients who died from medical errors is more than double the findings in a 1999 report that sparked widespread concern. The numbers in the new study are being challenged, but the findings promise to fuel the debate over hospital safety. The study by Health Grades Inc., a health-care consulting firm in Colorado that rates hospitals, estimated that medical errors in U.S. hospitals contributed to almost 600,000 patient deaths over the past three years, double the number of deaths from a study published in 2000 by the Institute of Medicine."

Laura Landro, "Report Card to Rank Hospitals on Safety," *Wall Street Journal*, 22 April 2004. "The incidence of medical errors is higher than some patients might think. The Institute of Medicine reported in 2000 that medical errors cause as many as 98,000 deaths annually, but some safety experts now say the report actually understates the problem. Charles Denham, a physician and founder of the nonprofit Texas Medical Institute of Technology, which designed the new survey [for reporting hospital safety], says a more realistic number may be as high as 200,000 deaths per year. . . . He says, 'the risk to patients is so great that we just don't have time to wait.'"

"Estimates of Healthcare-Associated Infections," Centers for Disease Control and Prevention, http://www.cdc.gov/ncidod/dhqp/hai.html, 15 June 2009. "In American hospitals alone, healthcare-associated infections account for an estimated 1.7 million infections and 99,000 associated deaths each year."

Jeff Donn, "Experts Warn on Expense of U.S. Drugs," *Associated Press*, 17 April 2005. "Well over 125,000 Americans die from drug reactions and mistakes each year, according to Associated Press projections from landmark medical studies of the 1990s. That could make pharmaceuticals the fourth-leading national cause of death after heart disease, cancer and stroke."

Saul Weingart, Ross McL. Wilson, Robert W. Gibberd, and Bernadette Harrison, "Epidemiology of Medical Error," *BMJ*, 18 March 2000. Adverse drug events among people not in hospitals "accounted for 116 million extra visits to the doctor per year, 76 million additional prescriptions, 17 million emergency department visits, 8 million admissions to [the] hospital, 3 million admissions to long term care facilities, and 199,000 additional deaths."

Laura Landro, "In the Hospital, Facing a Scourge of Killer Clots," *Wall Street Journal*, 01 April 2009. "Life-threatening blood clots are a growing problem in hospitals. . . . Deep-vein thrombosis, or DVT . . .

followed by pulmonary embolism — a sequence of occurrences known as a venous thromboembolism event, or VTE — kills nearly 200,000 U.S. patients a year." This condition is viewed as almost entirely preventable.

2. Christopher Lee, "Studies: Hospitals Could Do More to Avoid Infections — Poor Hygiene, Operating Room Traffic, Antibiotic Use Are Cited," *Washington Post*, 21 November 2006. "Infections acquired in hospitals, which take a heavy toll on patients, arise mainly from poor hygiene in hospital procedures, not from how sick patients were when they were admitted, according to three new studies." (Other researchers make similar points about medical errors and adverse drug events.)

3. The math for this calculation is derived from the calculation explained later in the chapter that 26% of deaths are directly caused by health care.

4. "Rank Order — Life Expectancy at Birth," *CIA World Factbook*, 19 March 2009, https://www.cia.gov/library/publications/the-world-factbook/rankorder/2102rank.html.

5. "Rank Order — Infant Mortality Rate," *CIA World Factbook*, 19 March 2009, https://www.cia.gov/library/publications/the-world-factbook/rankorder/2091rank.html. This analysis reports the country with the highest infant mortality rate as number one, so to derive rankings of the lowest infant mortality rate, one needs to start counting from the bottom of the list. I call this statistic "infant survival rates."

6. Nicholas D. Kristof, "Health Care? Ask Cuba," *New York Times*, 12 January 2005.

7. World Health Organization, "World Health Organization Assesses the World's Health Systems," 21 June 2000. An overview of the study can be found at http://www.who.int/whr/2000/media_centre/press_release/en/index.html. In the appendix, p. 13 provides the ranking showing the U.S. 37th overall: http://www.who.int/whr/2000/en/whr_annex_en.pdf. Some analysts object to the study's approach to ranking. Even if this study is discounted, dozens of others point in the same direction.

8. Paul Davies, "Fatal Medical Errors Said To Be More Widespread," *Wall Street Journal*, 27 July 2004. See also Laura Landro, "Report Card to Rank Hospitals on Safety," *Wall Street Journal*, 22 April 2004.

The story hasn't changed much since then. See "National Healthcare Quality Report 2008," U.S. Department of Health and Human Services, Agency for Healthcare Research and Quality, March 2009. It reports, "Distressingly, measures of patient safety . . . indicate not only a lack of improvement but also, in fact, a decline of almost 1 percent" in each of the most recent six years. This report can be found at www.ahrq.gov/qual/qrdr08.htm.

9. "Fourth Annual HealthGrades Patient Safety in American Hospitals Study: April 2007," Health Grades, Inc.

10. This is a subset of a list adapted from Linda T. Kohn, Janet M. Corrigan, and Molla S. Donaldson, eds., Institute of Medicine, *To Err is Human: Building a Safer Health System*, Washington: National Academies, 2000.

11. Kevin Sack, "Swabs in Hand, Hospital Cuts Deadly Infections," *New York Times*, 27 July 2007. See also "CDC Urges Hospitals to Tackle Drug-Resistant Infections," *Dow Jones Newswires*, 19 October 2006.

12. Wikipedia, "Ignaz Semmelweis," 10 June 2007, http://en.wikipedia.org/wiki/Ignaz_Semmelweis.

13. Christopher Lee, "Studies: Hospitals Could Do More to Avoid Infections — Poor Hygiene, Operating Room Traffic, Antibiotic Use Are Cited," *Washington Post*, 21 November 2006.

14. Robert Langreth, "Clean Hands," *Forbes.com*, 19 June 2006. "'Hand-washing can be the most powerful weapon on earth,' says New York University infection expert Philip M. Tierno, yet studies show doctors often forget to do it. . . . Strict infection-control measures and prudent antibiotic use have let hospitals in the Netherlands avoid the resistant staph strains that plague most U.S. hospitals. . . . Resis-

tant staph infections dropped 90% at the University of Pittsburgh Medical Center after it began testing incoming ICU patients for exposure to resistant staph strains and isolating carriers. . . . 'It saves money — and lives. There is no reason why this shouldn't be implemented in a universal way,' says Carlene Muto, head of infection control at the medical center."

See also Kevin Sack, "Swabs in Hand, Hospital Cuts Deadly Infections," *New York Times,* 27 July 2007.

15. Betsy McCaughey, "Coming Clean," *New York Times,* 06 June 2005.

16. Ibid.

17. Howard Gleckman with John Carey, "Medicine's Industrial Revolution," *Business Week,* 29 May 2006. "For 150 years we have known that doctors with unwashed hands pass infections from patient to patient. The Centers for Disease Control & Prevention figures that 80% of hospital-acquired infections are transmitted this way, costing billions of dollars annually to treat and killing thousands of people."

18. Liz Szabo, "Patient, Protect Thyself," *USA Today,* 04 February 2007. "Only about 35% of hospital employees consistently wash their hands each time they prepare to touch a patient — a basic step to preventing infection, O'Leary says." This quotation refers to Dennis O'Leary, who at the time headed the Joint Commission on Accreditation of Healthcare Organizations, which accredits hospitals.

19. Robert Langreth, "Fixing Hospitals," *Forbes,* 20 June 2005. A University of Geneva study (reported in *Annals of Internal Medicine*) noted, "61% of doctors wash their hands before examining a patient if they know someone is watching . . . 44% wash their hands if they think no one is watching."

20. Ahmedin Jemal, Rebecca Siegel, Elizabeth Ward, Yongping Hao, Jiaquan Xu, Taylor Murray, and Michael J. Thun, "Cancer Statistics, 2008," *CA — A Cancer Journal for Clinicians,* 20 February 2008. Total estimated deaths from breast cancer are 40,930.

21. Melonie P. Heron, Donna L. Hoyert, Jiaquan Xu, Chester Scott, and Betzaida Tejada-Vera, "Deaths: Preliminary Data for 2006," *National Vital Statistics Reports,* 11 June 2008. It noted that 44,572 people died as a result of motor vehicle accidents.

22. Laura Landro, "In the Hospital, Facing a Scourge of Killer Clots," *Wall Street Journal,* 01 April 2009. See also the website www.PreventDVT.org. Unless otherwise noted, the information in this section comes from these two sources.

23. Ibid.

24. Gina Maiocco, "DVT Prevention for the Obese Patient: Evidence-Based Nursing Interventions," *Bariatric Nursing and Surgical Patient Care,* 06 December 2008.

25. Jeff Donn, "Experts Warn on Expense of U.S. Drugs," *Associated Press,* 17 April 2005.

See also Saul Weingart, et al., "Epidemiology of Medical Error," *BMJ,* 18 March 2000.

26. Committee on Identifying and Preventing Medication Errors, Philip Aspden, Julie Wolcott, J. Lyle Bootman, Linda R. Cronenwett, eds., Institute of Medicine, *Preventing Medication Errors,* Washington: National Academies, 2006. A summary appears at http://www.iom.edu/Object.File/Master/35/943/medication%20errors%20new.pdf.

27. Thomas A. Sharon, *Protect Yourself in the Hospital: Insider Tips for Avoiding Hospital Mistakes for Yourself or Someone You Love,* Chicago: McGraw-Hill, 2003.

28. Gail Van Kanegan and Michael Boyette, *How to Survive Your Hospital Stay: The Complete Guide to Getting the Care You Need — and Avoiding Problems You Don't,* New York: Fireside, 2006.

29. Barbara Starfield, "Is US Health Really the Best in the World?" *JAMA,* 26 July 2000. The author explains her methodology for calculating deaths caused by health care, and concludes, "In any case,

225,000 deaths per year constitutes the third leading cause of death in the United States, after deaths from heart disease and cancer. Even if these figures are overestimated, there is a wide margin between these numbers of deaths and the next leading cause of death (cerebrovascular disease)."

See also "Deaths/Mortality" as reported by the federal government at: http://www.cdc.gov/nchs/fastats/deaths.htm. The top three causes of death and numbers of people who died of each in 2006 were:

- Heart disease   631,636
- Cancer   559,888
- Stroke (cerebrovascular diseases)   137,119

See also Timothy J. Mullaney, "Business, Heal Health Care," *Business Week*, 14 August 2006. "It's no secret how messy the U.S. health-care industry is. Americans spend 16% of gross domestic product on health care, but quality is poor. Medical mistakes are the nation's third-leading killer."

30. The figure of 624,000 deaths from health care gone awry discussed earlier in the chapter exceeds the 560K deaths from cancer, noted above, making health care the second leading cause of death in the United States. This figure is also nearly as great as the 632K deaths noted above for heart disease. As a result, health care is close to tying for first place as the leading cause of death in America.

31. Linda T. Kohn, Janet M. Corrigan, and Molla S. Donaldson, eds., Institute of Medicine, *To Err is Human: Building a Safer Health System*, Washington: National Academies, 2000.

32. Don Berwick's Institute for Healthcare Improvement (http://www.ihi.org/ihi/about) is seen by many to be leading the charge. See his book *Escape Fire* (Jossey-Bass, 2003) for his extraordinarily moving speeches at his annual convention — which today draws 6,000 health care professionals in person and thousands more via video link — focused on reducing the harm health care does to patients. An exceptionally humble and quietly spiritual man, Dr. Berwick breaks into tears talking about the tragedies caused by health care missteps.

See also Newt Gingrich with Dana Pavey and Anne Woodbury, *Saving Lives & Saving Money: Transforming Health and Healthcare*, Washington, D.C.: The Alexis de Tocqueville Institution, 2003. This book highlights the fact that high quality care is often far less expensive than poor quality care.

33. Lucian Leape and Karen Davis, "To Err Is Human; To Fail to Improve Is Unconscionable," *Commonwealth Fund*, 16 August 2005.

34. Kevin Sack, "Government Reports Criticize Health Care System," *New York Times*, 07 May 2009.

35. For this reason, these endnotes sometimes reference earlier research, which at times is more comprehensive in scope than are later updates. The later analysis often reports essentially the same conclusions.

36. Laura Landro, "Hospitals Put the Squeeze on Infection-Prevention Efforts," *Wall Street Journal*, 09 June 2009.

37. Ashish K. Jha and Arnold M. Epstein, "Hospital Governance and the Quality of Care," *Health Affairs*, online 06 November 2009.

38. "List of United States Cities by Population," Wikipedia, 21 June 2009, http://en.wikipedia.org/wiki/List_of_United_States_cities_by_population. Boston's population is listed as 608,352 as of 2007.

39. "Births, Marriages, Divorces and Deaths: Provisional Data for 2007," *CDC National Vital Statistics Reports*, 14 July 2008.

40. "September 11, 2001 Attacks," Wikipedia, 13 Dec 2009, http://en.wikipedia.org/wiki/September_11_attacks. Reportedly, 2,995 people died.

41. Icasualties.org, downloaded from http://icasualties.org/Iraq/index.aspx on 20 March 2009. U.S. military deaths to date were 4,260.

42. Elizabeth A. McGlynn, Steven M. Asch, John Adams, Joan Keesey, Jennifer Hicks, Alison DeCristofaro, and Eve A. Kerr, "The Quality of Health Care Delivered to Adults in the United States," *New England Journal of Medicine*, 26 June 2003.

43. Saul Weingart, Ross McL. Wilson, Robert W. Gibberd, and Bernadette Harrison, "Epidemiology of Medical Error," *BMJ*, 18 March 2000. This study also notes that outpatient adverse drug events result in 116 million extra visits to the doctor and 76 million additional prescriptions.

44. Jerald Winakur, "What Are We Going To Do With Dad?" *Health Affairs*, July/August 2005.

45. Ibid.

46. Donald M. Berwick, "Mont Sainte-Victoire," plenary speech at the Institute for Healthcare Improvement's 18th Annual National Forum on Quality Improvement in Health Care, 12 December 2006, references the "NCC-MERP" Framework. Source: Index of the National Coordinating Council for Medication Error Reporting and Prevention, http://www.nccmerp.org/pdf/indexColor2001-06-12. It appears that this framework was initially developed to categorize adverse drug events and other medication-related issues. Berwick appears to apply this classification more broadly to medical errors.

47. Ibid.

48. Ibid. Note that Berwick reports that 3% of the injuries fall into Category G, and 1% fall into Category I. By this estimate, 4% of the 15 million people harmed, or 600,000 people a year, are either permanently injured or killed as a result of the care they receive in U.S. hospitals.

49. Ibid.

50. Found at http://wwwonl.gov/sci/techresources/Human_Genome/medicine/medicine.shtml, 18 June 2007.

51. Heather S. Oliff, "Astonishing Advances in Tissue Regeneration," *Life Extension*, March 2006, http://www.lef.org/magazine/mag2006/mar2006_report_regen_02.htm.

52. *American Heritage Dictionary of the English Language, Fourth Edition*, Boston: Houghton Mifflin, 2000.

53. *The Free Dictionary.com*, http://medical-dictionary.thefreedictionary.com/nosocomial.

Chapter Two: Actions Speak Louder than Words

54. Ceci Connolly, "U.S. 'Not Getting What We Pay For,'" *Washington Post*, 30 November 2008. "As much as half of the $2.3 trillion spent today [on health care in the U.S.] does nothing to improve health."

Brent James, Vice President for Medical Research and Executive Director of the Institute for Healthcare Delivery Research, Intermountain Healthcare, in an address at the 4th Annual World Health Care Congress, 23 April 2007, on "Transformative IT": "32% of care provided is inappropriate. Over 50% of spending is waste."

Peter Lee, President and CEO, Pacific Business Group on Health, in an address at the 4th Annual World Health Care Congress, 23 April 2007 on "Transparency and Public Reporting on the Quality and Cost of Care": "We've seen data that suggests that 50% of care is wasted."

Julie Appleby, "Consumer Unease with U.S. Health Care Grows," *USA Today*, 16 October 2006. "Overuse and waste can include unnecessary treatments, tests repeated because original results were misplaced or reliance on ineffective treatments. 'Several credible estimates have come up with around 30% of health care is unnecessary,' says Richard Deyo, professor of medicine at the University of Washington in Seattle."

Gilbert M. Gaul, "Bad Hospitals Net More Money," *Washington Post*, 24 July 2005. "Researchers at Dartmouth Medical School, who have been studying Medicare's performance for three decades, estimate that as much as $1 of every $3 is wasted on unnecessary or inappropriate care. Other analysts put the figure as high as 40 percent."

55. Donald M. Berwick, "Less Is More . . . And Better," *Newsweek*, 16 October 2006. "What best predicts the rate [of certain surgical procedures] is the number of specialists per capita. The more doctors, the more doctor visits. The more hospital beds, the more days spent in the hospital . . . For many procedures, the variation is stunning. Compared with the lowest-use areas, people in the highest-use areas get 10 times as many prostate operations, six times as many back surgeries, seven times as many coronary angioplasties."

John Carey, "Smarter Patients, Cheaper Care," *Business Week*, 22 June 2009. "'There is good reason to believe 30% to 40% of what we are spending goes for unnecessary services and inefficient care,' says Dr. Elliott S. Fisher, director of the Center for Health Policy Research at Dartmouth Medical School."

56. Stephanie Saul, "Need a Knee Replaced? Check Your Zip Code," *New York Times*, 11 June 2007.

57. Reed Abelson, "Heart Procedure is Off the Charts in an Ohio City," *New York Times*, 18 August 2006.

58. Ibid.

59. Donald M. Berwick, "Less Is More . . . And Better," *Newsweek*, 16 October 2006.

60. On a related note, see "Practice Patterns, Not Patient Needs, Drive Medical Decisions and Cost," Robert Wood Johnson Foundation Content Alerts, 27 May 2009.

61. "Supply-Sensitive Care," The Dartmouth Atlas Project Topic Brief, downloaded 20 June 2007, http://www.dartmouthatlas.org/topics/supply_sensitive.pdf. "Patients . . . in high-spending areas had 82 percent more physician visits, 26 percent more imaging exams, 90 percent more diagnostic tests and 46 percent more minor surgery. Compared to low-intensity regions, patients with hip fractures, colon cancer and heart attacks . . . in high-intensity regions had higher mortality rates and worse 'scorecards' on measures of quality." It should be noted that most of these studies concern Medicare patients. Said another way, they are all insured and have very similar coverage.

62. Barry Meier, "New Effort Reopens a Medical Minefield," *New York Times*, 7 May 2009.

63. Institute of Medicine, "Fact Sheet 5. Uninsurance Facts and Figures," downloaded 22 June 2007, http://www.iom.edu/CMS/17645.aspx.

64. "Supply-Sensitive Care," The Dartmouth Atlas Project Topic Brief, downloaded 20 June 2007, http://www.dartmouthatlas.org/topics/supply_sensitive.pdf.

See also http://www.dartmouthatlas.org/press/2006_atlas_press_release.shtm. This press release reports on a Dartmouth study of 4.7 million Medicare patients which reports that, in many cases, more services and higher spending were associated with worse health outcomes compared to similar patients who received fewer services: "Hospitals that treat patients more intensively and spent more Medicare dollars did not get better results. Similarly, the regions with the best quality and outcomes used fewer resources relative to their high-cost counterparts."

See also John Carey, "When More Medicine Is Less," *Business Week*, 29 May 2006. "Getting more medical care, and paying more for it, can actually make your health worse."

See also Shannon Brownlee, "Putting Consumers in the Driver's Seat?" AHIP Coverage, 31 May 2005. "In fact, according to a recent study published in the *Annuals of Internal Medicine*, mortality in high-cost regions appears to be about two to five percent higher than in the lowest cost regions of the country. The most likely explanation for this is that elderly people who live in high-cost regions spend more time in hospitals than citizens in low-cost regions, and hospitals are risky places, where patients are exposed to the possibility of medical errors, drug interactions, and life-threatening infections."

65. Brian E. Kouri, R. Gregory Parsons, and Hillel R. Alpert, "Physician Self-Referral for Diagnostic Imaging: Review of the Empiric Literature," *American Journal of Roentgenology*, October 2002. "Nonra-

diologists performing their own imaging are at least 1.7 - 7.7 times as likely to order imaging as non-self-referring physicians in the same specialty who see patients with the same problems."

66. Sandeep Jauhar, "Many Doctors, Many Tests, No Rhyme or Reason," *New York Times*, 11 March 2008.

67. Gina Kolata, "10 Million Women Who Lack A Cervix Still Get Pap Tests," *New York Times*, 23 June 2004. "As many as 10 million women who have had hysterectomies and who no longer have a cervix are still getting Pap tests, a new study finds. . . . No professional organization recommends Pap tests for most women without a cervix. . . . 'These women are being screened for cancer in an organ that they don't have.'" The original research to which the article refers is Brenda E. Sirovich and H. Gilbert Welch, "Cervical Cancer Screening Among Women Without a Cervix," *JAMA*, June 2004. This article renders the number "almost" ten million, and this is the number I have noted in the text.

68. Ibid.

69. Ibid. The *New York Times* article notes the problem of false positives: "When a woman does not have a cervix, a doctor scrapes cells from her vagina instead, sending them off to be examined. And that, cancer experts say, is problematic. Vaginal cancer is exceedingly rare, and tests of vaginal cells are much more likely to result in false positives than they are to find vaginal cancers. A result is unnecessary vaginal biopsies that can result in their own false positives. As a result, women can end up having vaginal tissue removed to treat a cancer that is not even present."

70. "Alternative Diagnosis," www.wrongdiagnosis.com, downloaded 05 Mar 2009. "Misdiagnosis can and does occur and is reasonably common with error rates ranging from 1.4% in cancer biopsies to a high 20-40% misdiagnosis rate in emergency or ICU care. Surveys of patients also indicate the chance of experiencing a misdiagnosis to range from 8% to 40%."

71. Anahad O'Connor, "Deaths Go Unexamined and the Living Pay the Price," *New York Times*, 02 March 2004.

72. Lucian L. Leape, "Error in Medicine," *JAMA*, 21 December 1994.

73. David Leonhardt, "Why Doctors So Often Get It Wrong," *New York Times*, 22 February 2006.

74. Atul Gawande, *Complications: A Surgeon's Notes on an Imperfect Science*, New York: Henry Holt, 2002.

75. David E. Newman-Toker and Peter J. Pronovost, "Diagnostic Errors — The Next Frontier for Patient Safety," *JAMA*, 11 March 2009.

76. "Diagnostic Error: Is Overconfidence the Problem?" *American Journal of Medicine* Supplement, May 2008.

77. Gary Kantor, "Guest Software Review: Isabel Diagnosis Software," *HIStalk*, 31 January 2006.

78. Ibid. See also the website for Isabel Healthcare at www.isabelhealthcare.com/home/default.

79. David Leonhardt, "Why Doctors So Often Get It Wrong," *New York Times*, 22 February 2006.

Chapter Three: "Enough about me. Let's talk about you. What do *you* think of me?"

80. Others draw the same conclusion. See for example, Steven Pearlstein, "Fixing Health Care Starts With the Doctors," *Washington Post*, 12 July 2009: "At the end of the day . . . it is physicians who have the greatest impact on the cost and quality of health care we get. It is the docs who drive the decisions on what tests are ordered up, what surgeries performed and what drugs prescribed. And it is around the doctors and their practices that the medical system is organized."

81. Elizabeth A. McGlynn, Steven M. Asch, John Adams, Joan Keesey, Jennifer Hicks, Alison DeCristofaro, and Eve A. Kerr, "The Quality of Health Care Delivered to Adults in the United States,"

New England Journal of Medicine, 26 June 2003. All statistics in this paragraph are drawn from this article.

82. All quotations from Elizabeth A. McGlynn, et al., "The Quality of Health Care Delivered to Adults in the United States," *New England Journal of Medicine*, 26 June 2003.

83. Ibid.

84. "Most Americans Don't Get Preventive Healthcare," *Reuters Health*, 22 May 2006.

85. Ellen Nolte and C. Martin McKee, "Measuring the Health of Nations," *Health Affairs*, January/February 2008.

86. Ann M. Simmons, "Giving Parents a Dose of Confidence," *Los Angeles Times*, 20 May 2004.

87. Josee Rose, "Dose of Health 'Literacy' Helps Parents Avoid Trips to the ER," *Wall Street Journal*, 27 April 2004.

88. Ibid.

89. "Health, United States, 2008," U.S. Department of Health and Human Services, National Center for Health Statistics, 2009. Available at http://www.cdc.gov/nchs/hus.htm.

90. "Ten Great Public Health Achievements — United States, 1900-1999," *Morbidity and Mortality Weekly Report*, Centers for Disease Control, 02 April 1999. "During the 20th century, the health and life expectancy of persons residing in the United States improved dramatically. Since 1900, the average lifespan of persons in the United States has lengthened by greater than 30 years; 25 years of this gain are attributable to advances in public health."

See also James W. Henderson, *Health Economics and Policy*, Cincinnati: South-Western, 1999, p. 142. "Research on the relationship between health status and medical care frequently has found that the marginal contribution of medical care to health status is rather small."

See also Sherman Folland, Allen Goodman, and Miron Stano, *The Economics of Health and Health Care*, third edition, Upper Saddle River: Prentice Hall, 2001, p. 118. "The historical declines in population mortality rates were not due to medical interventions because effective medical interventions became available to populations largely after the mortality had declined. Instead, public health, improved environment, and improved nutrition probably played substantial roles."

91. *American Heritage Dictionary of the English Language, Fourth Edition*, New York: Houghton Mifflin, 2000. Public health is "The science and practice of protecting and improving the health of a community, as by preventive medicine, health education, control of communicable diseases, application of sanitary measures, and monitoring of environmental hazards."

92. "Health, United States, 2008," U.S. Department of Health and Human Services, National Center for Health Statistics, November 2008. Table 26.

93. Mitchell L. Cohen, "Changing Patterns of Infectious Disease," *Nature*, 17 August 2000. "For most of the twentieth century, the predominant feeling about the treatment, control and prevention of infectious diseases was optimism. In 1931, Henry Sigerist wrote[1], 'Most of the infectious diseases . . . have now yielded up their secrets . . . Many illnesses . . . had been completely exterminated; others had [been brought] largely under control.' Between 1940 and 1960, the development and successes of antibiotics and immunizations added to this optimism, and in 1969, Surgeon General William H. Stewart[2] told the United States Congress that it was time to 'close the book on infectious diseases.'" [Footnotes within the footnote can be found in the citation itself.]

94. "Health, United States, 2008," U.S. Department of Health and Human Services, National Center for Health Statistics, November 2008. Table 26.

95. "Chronic Disease Overview," Centers for Disease Control and Prevention at http://www.cdc.gov/nccdphp/overview.htm, downloaded 17 August 2009.

See also "Improving the Health and Quality of Life of All People," Centers for Disease Control and Prevention, http://www.cdc.gov/nccdphp/publications/brochure/brochure.htm, 15 November 2005 (link no longer functional). "Many of the actual causes of death in the United States are directly related to behavior choices such as tobacco use, poor nutrition, and physical inactivity."

See also Robert Langreth, "Just Say No," Forbes.com, 19 November 2004. "Epidemiological studies have found that bad living—smoking, drinking too much alcohol, feasting on cheeseburgers—is responsible for 80% of one's risk of heart disease and almost all of the risk of diabetes."

96. "Improving the Health and Quality of Life of All People," Centers for Disease Control and Prevention, http://www.cdc.gov/nccdphp/publications/brochure/brochure.htm, 15 November 2005 (link no longer functional). "Medical care for people with chronic diseases accounts for more than 75% of the $1.4 trillion that the United States spends each year on health care. . . . With the percentage of Americans over the age of 65 expected to double over the next 30 years, we cannot afford the escalating costs of health care. Many think that if we get better technology and more clinical care, we will solve these problems; however, past experience suggests we must balance our prevention and treatment efforts. If we are serious about improving the health and quality of life of all Americans and keeping our health care spending under control, we must commit to a national health agenda that supports prevention for every American. . . . Despite the proven benefits of physical activity and a healthy diet, more than 50% of American adults do not get the recommended amount of physical activity to provide health benefits, and only about 25% of U.S. adults eat the recommended five or more servings of fruits and vegetables each day."

See also Kathleen Fackelmann, "Stress Can Ravage The Body, Unless The Mind Says No," USA Today, 22 March 2005. "Up to 90% of the doctor visits in the USA may be triggered by a stress-related illness, says the Centers for Disease Control and Prevention. . . . A positive outlook on life and the support of friends might help buffer a damaging stress response."

See also Robert Langreth, "Just Say No," Forbes.com, 19 November 2004.

97. "U.S. Residents' Doctor Visits Increased Between 1994, 2004, CDC Study Finds," Kaiser Daily Health Policy Report, 26 June 2006. "Findings show that 1.1 billion doctor visits took place in 2004." Assuming a population of 300 million people, these figures mean that people visit the doctor on average 3.67 times each year.

98. S. Jay Olshansky, Douglas J. Passaro, Ronald C. Hershow, Jennifer Layden, Bruce A. Carnes, Jacob Brody, Leonard Hayflick, Robert N. Butler, David B. Allison, and David S. Ludwig, "A Potential Decline in Life Expectancy in the United States in the 21st Century," New England Journal of Medicine, 17 March 2005. In summary, the authors suggest that trends in levels of obesity presage a higher incidence of diabetes and concomitant reduced life expectancy.

See also "Obesity Threatens to Cut U.S. Life Expectancy, New Analysis Suggests," National Institutes of Health, 17 March 2005. "Over the next few decades, life expectancy for the average American could decline by as much as 5 years unless aggressive efforts are made to slow rising rates of obesity, according to a team of scientists supported in part by the National Institute on Aging (NIA), a component of the National Institutes of Health (NIH) of the Department of Health and Human Services (DHHS). The U.S. could be facing its first sustained drop in life expectancy in the modern era, the researchers say."

See also the 2008 video at www.healthiestnation.org, which notes, "For the first time our children will have shorter life expectancies than ours."

99. N. R. Kleinfield, "Diabetes and Its Awful Toll Quietly Emerge as a Crisis," New York Times, 09 January 2006.

100. Ibid.

101. Elizabeth Svoboda, "To Prevent Amputations, Doctors Call for Aggressive Care," *New York Times*, 07 November 2006.

102. Ibid.

103. Barnaby J. Feder, "New Priority: Saving Feet Of Diabetics," *New York Times*, 30 August 2005. One health organization is "sending them home with a new $150 device that makes it easy to check the skin temperature on the bottom of their feet every day, along with instructions to phone immediately if either foot is warmer than 90 degrees or if one foot is 4 degrees warmer than the other. Either reading is an early warning sign that an ulcer is developing."

104. Elizabeth Svoboda, "To Prevent Amputations, Doctors Call for Aggressive Care," *New York Times*, 07 November 2006.

105. Barnaby J. Feder, "New Priority: Saving Feet Of Diabetics," *New York Times*, 30 August 2005.

106. Gina Kolata, "Study Says Chatty Doctors Forget Patients," *New York Times*, 26 June 2007. The article goes on to say, "Four out of five times when a doctor interjected personal information, the doctor never returned to the topic under discussion before the interruption."

107. Ibid.

108. William Grimes, "Eating My Spinach: Four Days on the Uncle Sam Diet," *New York Times*, 23 January 2005.

109. Ibid.

110. Lauran Neergaard, "Moving Nation from Sick Care Toward Wellness Care," *Daily Courier*, 03 March 2009. "The doctor says, 'Lose weight, exercise, see you in a year.' We know that doesn't work." The speaker is the doctor in charge of integrative medicine at Duke University Medical Center.

111. Shari Roan, "Weight Loss: Why It's Hard," *Los Angeles Times*, 02 June 2008.

112. David Leonhardt, "Fat Tax," *New York Times*, 16 August 2009.

113. *American Heritage Dictionary of the English Language, Fourth Edition*, New York: Houghton Mifflin, 2000.

114. David Shore, remarks at the 2nd Annual Consumer-Centric Healthcare Congress, November 2006.

115. *American Heritage Dictionary of the English Language, Fourth Edition*, New York: Houghton Mifflin, 2000.

Chapter Four: The Patient as Footnote

116. Chuck Fager, Director, Quaker House, e-mail to the author, 12 June 2008.

See also Alfred McCoy, *A Question of Torture*, New York: Henry Holt, 2006. Prisoners held for interrogation may be subjected to either sensory deprivation or sensory overload. The effect is similar.

The fact that the characteristics listed are also representative of a hospital ICU was confirmed in dozens of conversations with hospital administrators, nurses, and doctors.

See also "Study: Lack of Sleep Hurts ICU Patients," *FierceHealthcare*, 18 December 2007, which summarizes a study that concluded in part, "Patient sleep is frequently disrupted by excessive light and noise, a lack of cues as to time of day . . . "

117. Ibid. Terrorist suspects may be drugged when in transit from one location to another, but are not typically drugged while being held for interrogation.

118. MedicineNet.com, downloaded 18 June 2008.

119. Ibid.

120. Ibid.

121. This is what the doctor treating a relative said to me, and this general response is confirmed by the following description in an article by Laura Landro, "Hospitals Combat an Insidious Complication," *Wall Street Journal*, 17 October 2007: "When someone is in the hospital, it is common to get confused and delirious, but the tradition in medicine has been to say, 'Don't worry if Grandma or Grandpa is confused, it's no big deal' . . . But it is a major public-health problem that has to be addressed."

122. Laura Landro, "Hospitals Combat an Insidious Complication," *Wall Street Journal*, 17 October 2007.

123. Gina Kolata, "A Tactic to Cut I.C.U. Trauma: Get Patients Up," *New York Times*, 12 January 2009. "Researchers say they are alarmed by what they are finding as they track patients for months or years after an I.C.U. stay. Patients, even young ones, can be weak for years. Some have difficulty thinking and concentrating or have post-traumatic stress disorder and terrible memories of nightmares they had while heavily sedated."

124. Laura Landro, "Hospitals Combat an Insidious Complication," *Wall Street Journal*, 17 October 2007. This conclusion is based on anecdotal evidence at the moment. However, the anecdotal evidence is strong. "Preliminary evidence shows that each day spent in a delirious state [another description for ICU Psychosis] increases the risk of long-term cognitive impairment by 35%. While many factors can contribute to such impairment, several studies have shown links between delirium, declining mental function and eventual dementia, says Dr. Ely. Patients can end up 'in their own little hell,' he says, where they have trouble thinking straight or doing simple tasks like balancing a checkbook. The causes of so-called acquired long-term cognitive impairment after ICU stays are being investigated in two large studies funded by Veterans Affairs and the National Institutes of Health." The article tells of a busy mid-career professional whose IQ dropped from 145 before an ICU stay to 110 afterwards — a drop of nearly 25%. This 40-something woman was forced to retire from her job because she could no longer do it, "and an MRI scan showed atrophy in her brain similar to what might appear in an 80-year-old woman with dementia, the progressive and permanent loss of memory and cognition." Now imagine what life is like post-ICU for someone who started out with an average IQ.

125. Ibid.

126. Siri Carpenter, "Is Your Parent Over-Medicated?" *Prevention*, December 2008.

127. Ibid.

128. W. David McCoy, "Abundance of 'Cures' Brings Ills," *New York Times*, 11 June 2002. I include this story to show that this situation has been a problem for many years.

129. Jane E. Brody, "The 'Poisonous Cocktail' of Multiple Drugs," *New York Times*, 18 September 2007.

130. "Fast Facts," American Hospital Association, 07 November 2008, found at www.aha.org/aha/content/2008/pdf/fast_facts_2008.pdf.

131. "ACHE Poll Finds Emphasis on Renovation, Infection Control," *Modern Healthcare*, 24 July 2007. This article provides a related point: in this case, 67% of hospital CEOs who responded to a survey said they were offering single-patient rooms, and the reason was to help control infections.

132. Laura Landro, "Hospitals Build a Better 'Healing Environment,'" *Wall Street Journal*, 21 March 2007.

See also "Hospital Room Design Can Have Effect on Patient Care, Outcomes, Studies Show," *Kaiser Daily Health Policy Report*, 19 May 2009.

See also Terri Cullen, "Putting 'Care' Back in Health Care," *Wall Street Journal*, 22 February 2007. The article is subtitled, "A Good Hospital Experience Makes Terri Wonder: Why Are Most Health-Care Providers So Aggravating?" The author discusses how poor much of the health care system is at treating patients as if it cares about them.

133. Andrea Hassol, James M. Walker, David Kidder, Kim Rokita, David Young, Steven Pierdon, Deborah Deitz, Sarah Kuck, and Eduardo Ortiz, "Patient Experiences and Attitudes about Access to a Patient Electronic Health Care Record and Linked Web Messaging," *Journal of the American Medical Informatics Association,* November/December 2004.

134. Robert G. Brooks and Nir Menachemi, "Physicians' Use of Email With Patients: Factors Influencing Electronic Communication and Adherence to Best Practices," *Journal of Medical Internet Research,* January - March 2006. "Among the physician-respondents, 2593 (63%) indicated the use of email from their office for communication with groups other than patients. Most commonly, they reported the use of email to communicate with friends or family members (74.2%), other doctors (63.8%), and for business-related communications (50.1%)."

See also "Internet Usage Statistics for North America," found at http://www.internetworldstats.com/am/us.htm, downloaded 06 March 2009.

135. "Many Physicians Do Not Use E-Mail to Communicate with Patients," *Kaiser Daily Health Policy Report,* 24 April 2008.

136. Andrea Hassol, James M. Walker, David Kidder, Kim Rokita, David Young, Steven Pierdon, Deborah Deitz, Sarah Kuck, and Eduardo Ortiz, "Patient Experiences and Attitudes about Access to a Patient Electronic Health Care Record and Linked Web Messaging," *Journal of the American Medical Informatics Association,* November/December 2004.

137. Ibid.

Chapter Five: The Mushroom Treatment

138. Surescripts website, http://www.surescripts.com/Surescripts/e-prescribing-facts.aspx#market, 27 February 2009. (link no longer functional). The following data was reported:

- 4,416,285,490 — Total Prescriptions Written
- 883,257,098 — Unfilled
- 3,533,028,392 — Total Dispensed
- The U.S. spent $270 billion on prescription drugs in 2007.

139. Ibid. 4,416,285,490 prescriptions written divided by 300 million people = 14.72/person.

140. "Taking Medicine Is an Important Part of Staying Healthy," *Aetna Member Essentials,* May 2009. This view is representative of the industry.

On a related note, there are entire businesses dedicated to helping pharmaceutical companies drive compliance. The website of one of these, Consumer Health Information Corporation, headlines its "Patient Compliance Strategies" section with the following comment: "The real measure of your product's success is how well you have convinced the patient to take your product correctly over the long term." In context, "correctly" appears to mean "takes all doses prescribed." Note that there is no reference to the idea that success might be measured in terms of improving patients' health.

141. Sundeep Khosla, "Increasing Options for the Treatment of Osteoporosis," *New England Journal of Medicine,* 12 August 2009.

142. Sandra G. Boodman, "Are Doctors To Blame?" *Washington Post,* 27 May 2008.

143. "Problems with Medical Decision-Making," *Foundation for Informed Medical Decision Making,* http://www.informedmedicaldecisions.org/problems_with_medical_decision_making.html, downloaded 17 October 2009.

144. Derjung M. Tarn, John Heritage, Debora A. Paterniti, Ron D. Hays, Richard L. Kravitz, and Neil S. Wenger, "Physician Communication When Prescribing New Medications," *Archives of Internal Medicine,* 25 September 2006.

145. This result is calculated by multiplying the six percentages listed. For those of you who are not statistics wizards, think of it this way: assume doctors tell 50 people out of 100 one fact. Then assume that you stand the same 100 people up in a row and the doctors tell a randomly chosen 50 of them a second fact. There's no reason to believe that the 50 people who heard the second fact are the same 50 people who heard the first fact. So it's logical to believe that the number of people who heard both facts is a lot less than 50. Mathematicians have figured out that it's likely to be 25 people who heard both facts. Another 25 heard neither fact, another 25 heard only the first fact, and another 25 heard only the second fact. When six facts are involved, it's clear that the number of people who hear all six facts is going to be very low unless the percent who hear each fact is very high — say, 95% or so. Even then, fewer than 75% of the people would have heard all six.

146. Duff Wilson, "Harvard Medical School in Ethics Quandary," *New York Times*, 04 March 2009.

147. Ibid.

One visible part of the medical school's response was a variation of "shoot the messenger" which one might term "muzzle the messenger." Shortly after the above *New York Times* article appeared, the school created a policy prohibiting any contact between students and the press that didn't go through the dean and the school's Public Affairs department, which deals with the press. After the entirely predictable outcry that this policy provoked, the school authorities appear to be recanting — in any event they promise to "revise" it. See Duff Wilson, "Harvard Backs Off Media Policy," *New York Times*, 02 September 2009.

148. Gardiner Harris, "Prosecutors Plan Crackdown on Doctors Who Accept Kickbacks," *New York Times*, 04 March 2009.

149. Ibid.

150. Gary Ahlquist, Charles Beever, Rick Edmunds, and David G. Knott, "Consumer and Physician Readiness for a Retail Healthcare Market: Changing the Basis of Competition," *Booz Allen Hamilton Consumerism Survey Report*, 2007.

151. Anne Harding, "Docs Often Write Off Patient Side Effect Concerns," *Reuters Health*, 28 August 2007.

152. Ibid.

153. Dr. Wall is an alias.

154. Susan Edgman-Levitan, "NQF 2008 Implementation Conference on Care Coordination: Communications," The John D. Stoeckle Center for Primary Care Innovation, March 2008.

Early underlying research: Clarence H. Braddock, III, Stephan D. Fihn, Wendy Levinson, Albert R. Jonsen, and Robert A. Pearlman, "How Doctors and Patients Discuss Routine Clinical Decisions," *Journal of General Internal Medicine*, June 1997. This research suggests that patients can be considered informed decision-makers if six characteristics are present in their conversation with the doctor: discussion of the decision to be made, discussion of alternatives, discussion of benefits and risks, discussion of uncertainties, assessing patients' understanding, and asking patients to express a preference. The study concludes that discussions about clinical decisions, on average, include only 1.23 of these. "Discussion of risks and benefits was less frequent (9%). The least frequently included element was discussion of the patient's degree of understanding (2%)." It does not appear that this picture has changed radically since this study was done.

155. This estimate is a synthesis of discussions with a variety of health care industry researchers. The most common views were that on average 40-50% of the time, any given individual is not helped by a given treatment.

156. "Lyrica Significantly Reduced Pain and Helped Patients Manage the Symptoms of Fibromyalgia, Data Show," *Pfizer press release*, 01 May 2007. "Significantly more patients treated with Lyrica reduced

their pain by 50 percent or more compared with placebo. Of those patients taking 600mg of Lyrica a day, 30 percent said their pain was cut in half or better; 27 percent of those taking 450mg a day and 24 percent of those taking 300mg also reported this level of pain relief. Of those taking placebo, 15 percent reported pain reduction of 50 percent or greater."

157. Lee Bowman, "New Diabetes Treatment Helped Prevent the Disease in Studies," *Topeka Capital-Journal*, 18 September 2006.

158. John Carey, "Do Cholesterol Drugs Do Any Good?" *Business Week*, 17 January 2008.

159. "Artificial Lumbar Disc Replacement," Blue Cross Blue Shield Technology Evaluation Center, 2007, http://www.bcbs.com/betterknowledge/tec/press/artificial-lumbar-disc.html, downloaded 24 June 2007.

160. Harry N. Herkowitz, "Total Disc Replacement with the CHARITE Artificial Disc Was as Effective as Lumbar Interbody Fusion," *Journal of Bone & Joint Surgery*, 01 May 2006. "Clinical success was defined as a ≥ 25% improvement in ODI [Oswestry Disability Index] score at 24 months [after surgery], no device failure, no major complications, and no neurological deterioration. . . . Clinical success was 64% in the Charite group."

161. John Carey, with Amy Barrett, "Is Heart Surgery Worth It?" *Business Week*, 18 July 2005.

162. John Carey, "Do Cholesterol Drugs Do Any Good?" *Business Week*, 17 January 2008. "The dramatic 36% figure has an asterisk. Read the smaller type. It says: 'That means in a large clinical study, 3% of patients taking a sugar pill or placebo had a heart attack compared to 2% of patients taking Lipitor.' Now do some simple math. The numbers in that sentence mean that for every 100 people in the trial, which lasted 3 1/3 years, three people on placebos and two people on Lipitor had heart attacks. The difference credited to the drug? One fewer heart attack per 100 people. So to spare one person a heart attack, 100 people had to take Lipitor for more than three years. The other 99 got no measurable benefit."

Researchers use a statistic called Number Needed to Treat (NNT) to clarify how many people have to take a drug for one person to benefit. In the previous example, the NNT is 100 — one hundred people had to take the drug for one person to benefit.

"For many other drugs, the NNTs are large. Take Avandia, GlaxoSmithKline's drug for preventing the deadly progression of diabetes. The blockbuster, with $2.6 billion in U.S. sales in 2006, made headlines in 2007 when an analysis of clinical trial data showed it increased the risk of heart attacks. The largely untold story: There's little evidence the drug actually helps patients. Yes, Avandia is very good at lowering blood sugar, just as statins lower cholesterol levels. But that doesn't translate into preventing the dire consequences of diabetes, including heart disease, strokes, and kidney failure. Clinical trials 'failed to find a significant reduction in cardiovascular events even with excellent glucose control,' wrote Dr. Clifford J. Rosen, chair of the Food & Drug Administration committee that evaluated Avandia, in a recent commentary in The New England Journal of Medicine. 'Avandia is almost the poster child for everything wrong with our system,' says UCLA's Hoffman. 'Its NNT is close to infinite.'"

On a related note, see Tara Parker-Pope, "A Call for Caution in the Rush to Statins," *New York Times*, 18 November 2008. She summarizes a study: "Only 1.8% of the subjects who took a placebo had a major cardiovascular problem during the study period. Among statin users, 0.9 percent did. In other words, the absolute risk of a serious cardiovascular problem (as opposed to the relative risk) was reduced by less than one percentage point."

NNT is explained further on a website, www.nntonline.net, run by Dr. Chris Cates. Dr. Cates has created a computer program to help doctors understand how to translate research results into more meaningful information to help them better practice medicine.

163. John Carey, "Do Cholesterol Drugs Do Any Good?" *Business Week*, 17 January 2008.

164. Leila Abboud, "Largest Ever Studies On Drugs for Depression, Schizophrenia Could Transform Treatment," *Wall Street Journal*, 27 July 2005.

165. "Prescription Drugs That Cause Weight Gain," *Johns Hopkins Health Alerts*, 23 January 2007, www.johnshopkinshealthalerts.com.

166. Charlene Laino, "Is Your Medicine Cabinet Making You Fat?" *WebMD Weight Loss Clinic*, 06 July 2007, downloaded from www.medicinenet.com.

167. Mary Duenwald, "Is Your Medicine Cabinet Making You Fat?" *New York Times*, 16 August 2005. Although two articles referenced in this section have the same headline, they are unrelated.

168. Kathleen Zelman, "Lose Weight, Gain Tons of Benefits," *webmd.com*, 23 June 2006. See also "Improving Your Health," U.S. Department of Health and Human Services, July 2006. "Losing 5 to 10 percent of your body weight can help improve your health."

169. Mary Duenwald, "Is Your Medicine Cabinet Making You Fat?" *New York Times*, 16 August 2005.

170. Ibid.

171. "Kaiser Health Tracking Poll," Kaiser Family Foundation, February 2009. When asked, "Do you currently take any prescription medicine on a daily basis, or not?" 49% said yes, 50% said no, and 1% declined to answer or did not know.

172. Orly Avitzur, "Be Wary of Narcotics to Treat Back Pain," *Consumer Reports*, May 2009.

173. Ibid.

174. Rahul K. Parikh, "Showing the Patient the Door, Permanently," *New York Times*, 10 June 2008.

175. Sean R. Tunis, "Reflections of Science, Judgment, and Value in Evidence-Based Decision-Making: A Conversation with David Eddy," *Health Affairs*, 19 June 2007.

176. John Carey, "Medical Guesswork," *Business Week*, 29 May 2006.

177. Ibid.

178. "Supply-Sensitive Care," A Dartmouth Atlas Project Topic Brief, *The Dartmouth Atlas of Health Care*, 15 January 2007. "There is unwarranted variation in the practice of medicine and the use of medical resources in the United States. There is underuse of effective care, misuse of preference-sensitive care, and overuse of supply-sensitive care."

"Effective care" tends to refer to low-tech prevention or maintenance protocols, such as blood sugar screening or having heart attack patients take aspirin to prevent a second heart attack. "Preference-sensitive care" refers to situations in which several viable treatment choices are available, and the decision should be the patient's, but often the doctor essentially makes a choice that is inconsistent with the patient's values and priorities. Health care policy experts term this discrepancy "misuse" of care. "Supply-sensitive care" refers to care for which the determining factor in the equation is not how sick the patient is nor how well they are likely to do after surgery, but how many specialists there are per 1000 patients in the geographic area.

179. Ibid.

180. Ibid. See also John Carey, "Smarter Patients, Cheaper Care?" *Business Week*, 22 June 2009. The article is subtitled, "Better-informed medical decisions could cut billions in health-care costs as patients opt for cheaper treatments."

See also Laura Landro, "Weighty Choices, in Patients' Hands," *Wall Street Journal*, 04 August 2009: "Studies show that when patients understand their choices and share in the decision-making process with their doctors, they tend to choose less-invasive and less-expensive treatments than they would have otherwise received."

181. Gina Kolata, "Medicare Says It Will Pay, but Patients Say 'No Thanks,'" *New York Times*, 03 March 2006.

182. "National Emphysema Treatment Trial (NETT): Evaluation of Lung Volume Reduction Surgery for Emphysema," Department of Health and Human Services, National Institutes of Health, National Heart, Lung, and Blood Institute, http://www.nhlbi.nih.gov/health/prof/lung/nett/lvrsweb.htm#results, 20 May 2003.

183. Gina Kolata, "Medicare Says It Will Pay, but Patients Say 'No Thanks,'" *New York Times*, 03 March 2006.

184. Ibid.

185. Annette M. O'Connor, Hilary A. Llewellyn-Thomas, and Ann Barry Flood, "Modifying Unwarranted Variations in Health Care: Shared Decision Making Using Patient Decision Aids," *Health Affairs*, 07 October 2004.

Chapter Six: "Keep Away"

186. "Keep Away" is a children's game in which a ball is thrown among players in a circle but deliberately kept from the one child in the center of the circle. See http://en.wikipedia.org/wiki/Keep_Away.

187. "The Public Needs to Understand the Uncertainty of Medicines Regulation," *Scrip*, 23 January 2006. These comments were made by Harry Cayton, U.K. Department of Health Director for Patients and the Public. While he is referring to the U.K., the situation is very similar in the U.S.

188. Steve Dunn, "Cancer Basics," http://cancerguide.org/basic.html, March 2009. "In general, stage I cancers are small localized cancers that are usually curable, while stage IV usually represents inoperable or metastatic cancer."

See also "Stages of Endometrial Cancer," http://www.nlm.nih.gov/medlineplus/ency/article/000910.htm, 02 May 2008.

189. Dr. Green is an alias.

Chapter Seven: Children's Table at Thanksgiving

190. "Patient Knowledge Lacking at Hospital Discharge," *Reuters Health*, 16 August 2005.

191. Maggie Van Ostrand, "Thanksgiving and the Little Table," *TexasEscapes.com* downloaded 04 March 2009.

192. Andrea Hassol, James M. Walker, David Kidder, Kim Rokita, David Young, Steven Pierdon, Deborah Deitz, Sarah Kuck, and Eduardo Ortiz, "Patient Experiences and Attitudes about Access to a Patient Electronic Health Care Record and Linked Web Messaging," *Journal of the American Medical Informatics Association*, November/December 2004.

Five years later, the story remains the same. See Liz Kowalczyk, "Patients to Get a Look at Physicians' Notes," *Boston Globe*, 19 June 2009, which reports: "Many doctors say they are uncomfortable with the idea of sharing their notes. Of course, patients have a legal right to obtain their paper records, which usually include notes, but they often have to wait months to get copies and must pay a fee. Online access would be easy and immediate."

193. M. L. Baker, "EHRs Enter Patient-Doctor Relationships," *eWeek*, 2 April 2006.

194. Working Group on Policies for Electronic Information Sharing Between Doctors and Patients, "Connecting Americans to Their Healthcare — Final Report," Markle Foundation, July 2004, p. 82.

195. Paul C. Tang and David Lansky, "The Missing Link: Bridging the Patient-Provider Health Information Gap," *Health Affairs*, September/October 2005.

196. Ibid. "A California law . . . requires additional physician and patient consent for patients to access their information electronically. This state law also says that certain results (for example, abnormal

Pap smears) may not be released electronically for any reason, regardless of a patient's request."

197. Information about your legal rights to your medical records and how to get them can be found at http://ihcrp.georgetown.edu/privacy/records.html.

198. Andrea Hassol, James M. Walker, David Kidder, Kim Rokita, David Young, Steven Pierdon, Deborah Deitz, Sarah Kuck, and Eduardo Ortiz, "Patient Experiences and Attitudes about Access to a Patient Electronic Health Care Record and Linked Web Messaging," *Journal of the American Medical Informatics Association,* November/December 2004. "Like paper-based records, EHRs can have problems with accuracy and completeness. In our study, approximately 65% of patients rated their personal health information as complete and approximately 75% of them rated their medical history as accurate."

199. Ibid.

200. "Alternative Diagnosis," www.wrongdiagnosis.com, downloaded 05 Mar 2009. "Misdiagnosis can and does occur and is reasonably common with error rates ranging from 1.4% in cancer biopsies to a high 20-40% misdiagnosis rate in emergency or ICU care. Surveys of patients also indicate the chance of experiencing a misdiagnosis to range from 8% to 40%."

See also Atul Gawande, *Complications: A Surgeon's Notes on an Imperfect Science,* New York: Henry Holt, 2002. p. 196 of the paperback edition: "How often do autopsies turn up a major misdiagnosis in the cause of death? . . . According to three studies . . . the figure is about 40 percent . . . in about a third of the misdiagnoses the patients would have been expected to live if proper treatment had been administered." He goes on to point out that there has been no improvement in diagnostic accuracy, as far as autopsies show, since at least 1938.

201. Paul C. Tang and David Lansky, "The Missing Link: Bridging the Patient-Provider Health Information Gap," *Health Affairs,* 13 September 2005.

202. Sharon Sung, "Direct Reporting of Laboratory Test Results to Patients by Mail to Enhance Patient Safety," *Journal of General Internal Medicine,* October 2006.

203. This is a rough calculation, derived from the following data:
- In 2006, about 213,000 women were newly diagnosed with breast cancer. U.S. Preventive Services Task Force, www.cancer.org/downloads/stt/CAFF06EsCsMc.pdf, 30 October 2006.
- About 66% of women over the age of 40 report getting mammograms at least once in the last two years. Rita Rubin, "More Women over 40 Skip Regular Mammograms," *USA Today,* 13 May 2007.
- There are about 67 million women over the age of 40. http://www.census.gov/population/www/socdemo/men_women_2004.html. I derived this number by adding up the number of women aged 45 and older and adding half the number of women aged 35-44. While the result is not going to be precisely correct, the difference is not significant for this calculation.

Assume that the 66% of women over the age of 40 who had mammograms in the last two years had only one mammogram in that time, so that the annual rate is half that, or 33%. This means that there were 67 million x 33% = roughly 22 million women who had mammograms, a probable understatement since many have them annually. Since there are 213,000 women newly diagnosed with breast cancer in the course of a year and at least 22 million who have mammograms, that means that more than 100 women have mammograms for every one diagnosed with breast cancer (22 million/213K). If the women in fact get mammograms every year, it would mean more than 200 people get screened for every one diagnosed.

204. The math is a little more complicated than this due to false positives, but that doesn't change the main point. For a discussion of false positives, see Michael Blastland and Andrew Dilnot, "When Numbers Deceive," *The Week,* 27 February 2009, an extract from their book *The Numbers Game.* Simplifying the story somewhat: about 8 women out of 100 would be told that they had cancer. In fact, 7 of these would be false positives. That means that 92 women would be relieved, and 8 should be told promptly, "We need to run another test."

205. Daniel Gilbert, "What You Don't Know Makes You Nervous," *New York Times*, 20 May 2009.

206. Ibid.

207. Gina Kolata, "Sick and Scared, and Waiting, Waiting, Waiting," *New York Times*, 20 August 2005.

208. Ibid. The article goes on to discuss the fact that doctors dismiss as unimportant and not fixable the fact that patients don't like waiting, when solutions are available.

209. Tara Parker-Pope, "Study Equates Stress of Cancer and of Wait for Biopsy Data," *New York Times*, 25 February 2009.

210. Ibid.

211. Melinda Beck, "Stress So Bad It Hurts — Really," *Wall Street Journal*, 17 March 2009.

212. Kathleen Fackelmann, "Stress Can Ravage the Body, Unless the Mind Says No," *USA Today*, 22 March 2005.

213. Ibid. See also Claudia Dreifus, "Finding Clues to Aging in the Fraying Tips of Chromosomes," *New York Times*, 03 July 2007. Psychological stress causes cells to age, and the aging of the cells is highly correlated with cardiovascular disease and may be correlated with cancer. It appears that stress literally ages people and directly causes many diseases.

214. Sharon Sung, "Direct Reporting of Laboratory Test Results to Patients by Mail to Enhance Patient Safety," *Journal of General Internal Medicine*, October 2006.

See also T.K. Gandhi, "Fumbled Handoffs: One Dropped Ball After Another," *Annals of Internal Medicine*, 01 March 2005. This study reports that doctors tell patients normal results only 25% of the time, and abnormal ones only 67% of the time.

215. Bill Hendrick, "Patients Not Always Told of Lab Results," *WebMD Health News*, 22 June 2009.

216. Ibid.

217. Sharon Sung, "Direct Reporting of Laboratory Test Results to Patients by Mail to Enhance Patient Safety," *Journal of General Internal Medicine*, October 2006.

218. Lawrence P. Casalino, Daniel Dunham, Marshall H. Chin, Rebecca Bielang, Emily O. Kistner, Theodore G. Karrison, Michael K. Ong, Urmimala Sarkar, Margaret A. McLaughlin, David O. Meltzer, "Frequency of Failure to Inform Patients of Clinically Significant Outpatient Test Results," *Archives of Internal Medicine*, 22 June 2009.

219. Michael K. Paasche-Orlow, Holly A. Taylor, and Frederick L. Brancati, "Readability Standards for Informed-Consent Forms as Compared with Actual Readability," *New England Journal of Medicine*, 20 February 2003.

220. Ibid.

221. "Health Literacy Overview," Columbia University School of Nursing, found at http://www.nursing.
columbia.edu/informatics/HealthLitRes/overview.html. Downloaded 17 August 2009.

222. "'What Did the Doctor Say?' Improving Health Literacy to Protect Patient Safety," *Joint Commission*, 2007.

223. Daniel R. Beyer, Michael S. Lauer, Steve Davis, "Letter to the Editor: Readability of Informed-Consent Forms," *New England Journal of Medicine*, 29 May 2003.

224. "Problems with Patient Communication Increase Risk for Injury, Death," *Kaiser Daily Health Policy Report*, 26 March 2007. This article describes a news article appearing in *USA Today* which summarizes a report published by the Joint Commission on Accreditation of Healthcare Organizations, which accredits hospitals.

225. "JCAHO Asks Clinicians to Speak Plain English," *FierceHealthcare*, 08 February 2007.

226. Marie Skelton, "Report: Patient Illiteracy Threatens Health Care," *USA Today*, 25 March 2007.

227. Jane Brody, "The Importance of Knowing what the Doctor is Talking about," *New York Times*, 30 January 2007.

228. Roy P. C. Kessels, "Patients' Memory for Medical Information," *Journal of the Royal Society of Medicine*, May 2003.

229. Ibid.

230. Ibid.

231. "Health Advocate: A Remedy for Healthcare Confusion," *PR Newswire*, 10 October 2006.

Chapter Eight: "I don't get no respect." "I can't get no satisfaction."

232. This quotation is commonly attributed to Theodore Roosevelt.

233. Professor Miller, now emeritus, was a tireless advocate for students. Drawing a parallel to the concept of "patient-centric" in health care, one might term him "student-centric" in education. He championed a focus on providing students with what they needed from the school in order to get the best outcomes. When my personal medical crisis struck, he was one of the first people to whom I turned for support. Even though the situation had nothing to do with academics, I recognized that he would take a student/patient/individual-centric view and think through what I needed to know in order to proceed. After the surgery, as my family sat in a waiting room, he somehow talked his way into the Intensive Care Unit and confirmed that my mental faculties were intact.

234. "Grasping for Straws," *Mystery Diagnosis*, Discovery Health Channel, Season 1, Episode 5, first aired 21 November 2005.

235. Jerome Groopman, *How Doctors Think*, Boston/New York: Houghton Mifflin, 2007. One of the cover blurbs comments, "Dr. Jerome Groopman lifts the veil on possibly the most taboo topic in medicine: the pervasive nature of misdiagnosis. His engrossing narrative exposes all of the subtle mental traps — the snap judgments and stereotypical thinking, the premature conclusions and herd instinct — that dangerously narrow the vision of too many physicians."

236. Ibid.

237. Ibid. The preceding paragraphs are drawn from Dr. Groopman's account of the patient's experience.

238. Rosemary Gibson and Janardan Prasad Singh, *Wall of Silence: The Untold Story of the Medical Mistakes That Kill and Injure Millions of Americans*, New York: Lifeline Press, 2003.

239. Ibid.

240. "Restless Legs Syndrome," Mayo Clinic, 17 August 2009.

241. This anecdote, complete with the man's name and comments from his widow, appeared in a publication by the Restless Legs Syndrome Foundation. When I was unable to locate the document, I spoke with several Board members of the organization, who commented that a number of people have killed themselves under similar circumstances as a result of undiagnosed RLS. The Summer 2009 issue of *Nightwalkers*, the organization's quarterly magazine, contains a short submission by a reader that echoes the experience of the patient described here. The writer notes that given more information about the condition, "Doctors no longer think I'm crazy!"

242. Robert Klitzman, "CASES: Seeing Risk and Reward Through a Patient's Eyes," *New York Times*, 27 May 2003.

243. Ibid. All quotations in this section are from this article.

244. Tony Miksanek, "On Caring for 'Difficult' Patients," *Health Affairs*, September/October 2008. The doctor's description of the three patients in this section comes from this article.

245. Howard Markel, "When Hospitals Kept Children From Parents," *New York Times*, 01 January 2008.

246. Melinda Beck, "Bedside Manner: Advocating for a Relative in the Hospital," *Wall Street Journal*, 28 October 2008, quoting Beverly Johnson, president of the Institute for Family-Centered Care.

247. Melinda Beck, "Bedside Manner: Advocating for a Relative in the Hospital," *Wall Street Journal*, 28 October 2008.

248. "MCG Health," Institute for Family Centered Care, http://www.familycenteredcare.org/prfiles/prof-mcg.html, downloaded 14 December 2009.

249. Laura Landro, "When a Hospital Let Families Call for Rapid-Response Help," *Wall Street Journal*, 31 August 2009.

250. Ibid.

251. Randolph Fillmore, "Hopkins And State Team Up On Bioethics," *Johns Hopkins Gazette*, 23 June 1997. "A quiet but stunning bomb dropped on the health care community in November 1995. That's when the SUPPORT Study, a Robert Wood Johnson Foundation $28 million multi-center study, found that in hospitals across the nation, despite the world's best medical care, the critically ill were not receiving the care they wanted and needed. Worse, the study disclosed that interventions aimed at improving the care of the dying, implemented in phase two of the study, had no effect as physicians continued to ignore advance directives, living wills and patient wishes."

252. Susan Gilbert, "Study Finds Doctors Refuse Patients' Requests on Death," *New York Times*, 22 November 1995.

253. See, for example, Joan M. Teno, Brian R. Clarridge, Virginia Casey, Lisa C. Welch, Terrie Wetle, Renee Shield, and Vincent Mor, "Family Perspectives on End-of-Life Care at the Last Place of Care," *JAMA*, 07 January 2004, which notes that about a quarter of families "reported concerns with physician communication regarding medical decision making."

Similarly, a description of Dr. Joseph S. Weiner's work found at http://www.northshorelij.com/body.cfm?1d=2719&oTopID=2719&PLinkID=2584, 04 February 2006, reports: "Approaching Death: Improving Care at the End-of-Life' summarized serious deficiencies in end-of-life patient care. These deficiencies include poor pain management, aggressive care counter to patients' wishes, and lack of physician training."

254. A video documenting classroom sessions and their effect on the students who went through the experience can be found at www.pbs.org/wgbh/pages/frontline/shows/divided/.

Chapter Nine: Torture

255. http://www.dannyhaszard.com/stockholm_syndrome.htm.

See also http://en.wikipedia.org/wiki/Stockholm_syndrome.

See also http://ask.yahoo.com/20030324.html. "It's important to note that these symptoms occur under tremendous emotional and often physical duress. The behavior is considered a common survival strategy for victims of interpersonal abuse, and has been observed in battered spouses, abused children, prisoners of war, and concentration camp survivors."

See also http://marriage.about.com/od/domesticviolence/g/stockholmsyn.htm. "Stockholm Syndrome is a common survival mechanism of . . . those in controlling and/or intimidating relationships."

See also http://serendip.brynmawr.edu/bb/neuro/neuro04/web1/kkrasnec.html. "This development occurs when there are perceived threats of violence, disempowerment of the subject, high levels of stress or trauma upon [the] subject, and ultimate dependence upon the person in control for base survival."

See also http://www.knut.com/english/stockhs.html. "It takes only 3-4 days for the characteristic bond of the Stockholm syndrome to emerge when captor and captive are strangers. After that, research shows, the duration of captivity is no longer relevant." Excerpted from Jeri Martinez, *Domestic Violence Response Training Curriculum*, November 1991.

See also Dee L.R. Graham, Edna Rawlings, and Nelly Rimini, "Survivors of Terror: Battered Women, Hostages, & The Stockholm Syndrome," in *Feminist Perspectives on Wife Abuse*, Kirsti Yllo and Michele Bograd, eds., Sage: Thousand Oaks, 1988. "Victims are encouraged to develop psychological characteristics pleasing to captors: submissiveness, passivity, docility, dependency, lack of initiative, inability to act, decide, think, etc."

See also Paul T. P. Wong, "Elizabeth Smart and the Stockholm Syndrome," *Interpersonal Network on Personal Meaning*, http://www.meaning.ca/archives/archive/art_stockhom-syndrome_P_Wong.htm, undated, downloaded 14 July 2007.

256. Paul T. P. Wong, "Elizabeth Smart and the Stockholm Syndrome," *Interpersonal Network on Personal Meaning*, http://www.meaning.ca/archives/archive/art_stockhom-syndrome_P_Wong.htm, undated, downloaded 14 July 2007.

257. "Stockholm Syndrome," undated, downloaded 14 July 2007 from http://www.knut.com/english/stockhs.html.

258. Laura Landro, "Finding a Way to Ask Doctors Tough Questions," *Wall Street Journal*, 04 March 2009.

259. Ibid.

260. Jon Harding, "The Penalty For Being Difficult," *Health Affairs*, January/February 2009.

261. Ibid.

262. Laura Landro, "Finding a Way to Ask Doctors Tough Questions," *Wall Street Journal*, 04 March 2009.

263. http://www.dannyhaszard.com/stockholm_syndrome.htm.

264. Dee L.R. Graham, Edna Rawlings, and Nelly Rimini, "Survivors of Terror: Battered Women, Hostages, & The Stockholm Syndrome," in *Feminist Perspectives on Wife Abuse*, Kirsti Yllo and Michele Bograd, eds., Sage: Thousand Oaks, 1988.

265. Donald M. Berwick, "What 'Patient-Centered' Should Mean: Confessions of an Extremist," *Health Affairs*, web exclusive, 19 May 2009.

Chapter Ten: Gods and Mortals

266. Esther Jansen, Sandra Mulkens and Anita Jansen, "Do Not Eat the Red Food!: Prohibition of Snacks Leads to Their Relatively Higher Consumption in Children," *Appetite*, November 2007. "In this study, it was tested whether a prohibition of food in the first phase would lead to an increase in desire for the target food and overeating in the second phase. Sure enough, desire increased significantly in the prohibition group, whereas it remained constant in the no-prohibition group."

Consider also Marije Nije Bijvank, Elly A. Konijn, Brad J. Bushman, and Peter H. M. P. Roelofsma, "Age and Violent-Content Labels Make Video Games Forbidden Fruits for Youth," *Pediatrics*, 03 March 2009. Classifying a game as appropriate for older users, for example, made it more attractive to young children.

Consider also Liz Plosser, "Got Cravings? Ditch That Diet Mentality," *MSNBC.com*, 23 May 2008, which notes, "Ever notice that when you decide to give up a favorite food, it's the only thing you can think about? You're totally normal. When researchers at the University of Toronto deprived women of chocolate for a week, they found that the restrained eaters experienced more intense, chronic chocolate cravings and swallowed approximately double the amount of the forbidden food when it was finally allowed."

Consider also "The Porn Paradox," *The Week*, 20 March 2009. "Guess which states are most interested in online pornography? That's right — those with the highest concentrations of politically conservative and traditionally religious people . . . Utah boasts the highest porn-buying rate in the entire nation." Why? "If you're told you can't have this, then you want it more."

267. Doctors, like the rest of us, are a mixed lot. Some doctors approach their patients' imminent deaths with compassionate support rather than with a flurry of high-tech interventions, and thus give a profound gift both to patients and to their families. This approach to care is described in a book written by Dennis McCullough, *My Mother, Your Mother: Embracing "Slow Medicine," the Compassionate Approach to Caring for Your Aging Loved One*, New York: Harper, 2008. Yet, as Dr. Cullough notes: "So often today . . . we face a medical care system that seems to work at odds with our parents' stated desires and wishes. . . . Stories of elders' and families' distress abound."

268. "John Dalberg-Acton, 1st Baron Acton," *Wikipedia*, downloaded 12 March 2009. Lord Acton was an historian in England in the 1800s.

269. Dacher Keltner, "The Power Paradox," *Greater Good*, Winter 2007-2008.

270. "Understanding Older Patients," *Talking with Your Older Patient: A Clinician's Handbook*, National Institute on Aging, October 2008, found at http://www.nia.nih.gov/HealthInformation/Publications/ClinicianHB/02_understanding.htm.

271. Paul Starr, *The Social Transformation of American Medicine: The Rise of a Sovereign Profession and the Making of a Vast Industry*, New York: Basic Books, 1982.

272. Diana B. Henriques and Jack Healy, "Madoff Goes to Jail After Guilty Pleas," *New York Times*, 13 March 2009.

273. Joe Nocera, "Madoff Had Accomplices: His Victims," *New York Times*, 14 March 2009.

274. Ibid.

275. "CMS Visions on Quality Standards," 4th Annual World Health Care Congress, Washington, DC, 23 April 2007. This panel discussion included a representative from the American Medical Association.

276. "Fewer Patients Using Health Care Provider Quality Ratings Web Sites To Make Decisions," *Kaiser Daily Health Policy Report*, 02 December 2008.

277. Laura Landro, "Learning to Ask Tough Questions of Your Surgeon," *Wall Street Journal*, 09 January 2008.

278. Laura Landro, "Finding a Way to Ask Doctors Tough Questions," *Wall Street Journal*, 04 March 2009.

279. Anne Harding, "Docs Often Write Off Patient Side Effect Concerns," *Reuters Health*, 28 August 2007.

280. Roni Caryn Rabin, "With Rise in Radiation Exposure, Experts Urge Caution on Tests," *New York Times*, 19 June 2007.

281. Alex Berenson, "Study Finds Radiation Risk for Patients," *New York Times*, 27 August 2009.

282. Roni Caryn Rabin, "With Rise in Radiation Exposure, Experts Urge Caution on Tests," *New York Times*, 19 June 2007.

283. Alex Berenson, "Study Finds Radiation Risk for Patients," *New York Times*, 27 August 2009.

284. Katharine Greider, "Dirty Hospitals," *AARP Bulletin*, January 2007, quoting Betty McCaughey, who founded the Committee to Reduce Infection Deaths.

285. Amy L. Pakyz, Conan MacDougall, Michael Oinonen, and Ronald E. Polk, "Trends in Antibac-

terial Use in US Academic Health Centers 2002 to 2006," *Archives of Internal Medicine*, 10 November 2008. "Antibacterial drug use is a major risk factor for bacterial resistance."

286. Nicholas Bakalar, "Antibiotic Use in First Year May Increase Asthma Risk," *New York Times*, 19 June 2007.

287. Apparently one of the leading causes of receding gums is repeated aggressive brushing of one's teeth. See "Receding Gums," *California Dental Association*, http://www.cda.org/popup/Receding_Gums, downloaded 23 July 2007.

See also http://en.wikipedia.org/wiki/Gum_recession.

288. "Wearing Helmets 'More Dangerous,'" *BBC News*, 11 September 2006.

289. Tara Parker-Pope, "Want Fat With That? A Surprising Way To Make Vegetables More Nutritious," *Wall Street Journal*, 08 August 2006.

290. Ibid.

291. Denise Mann, "Germs in the Kitchen," *WebMD*, originally posted in 2005, reviewed by the site 18 October 2007.

292. M.P. McQueen, "Wellness Plans Reach Out to the Healthy," *Wall Street Journal*, 03 April 2007. One employer "used to offer $250 to employees who could stay smoke-free for several months. But some workers took up smoking just so they could then quit and qualify for the reward."

293. Charles Duhigg, "Warning: Habits May Be Good for You," *New York Times*, 13 July 2008.

294. Ibid.

295. "Red-Light Cameras Increase Accidents: 5 Studies That Prove It," *National Motorists Association*, 08 January 2008. See also "Cameras Increase Fatal Rear End Accidents," *thenewspaper.com*, 29 March 2005.

296. "What To Do When Patients Lie," *FierceHealthcare*, 22 January 2007.

Similarly, Cathryn Gunther, health care strategist, e-mail to the author, 08 December 2009, notes that patients may be ashamed of their own less-than-stellar behavior. She concludes: "With so little time to establish a trusting relationship with individuals, physicians can create an environment where the patient feels more comfortable telling a fib, rather than the truth about their own behavior."

297. Carla K. Johnson, "Doctors Say Patients Who Lie May Put Their Health at Risk," *Associated Press*, 19 January 2007.

298. Ibid.

299. Ibid.

Chapter Eleven: There's Many a Slip 'Twixt the Cup and the Lip

300. The description of process steps related to a doctor's visit is adapted from Elizabeth L. Bewley, *Solving America's Health Care Problems*, 1996. That white paper is available for free download at http://www.pariohealth.net/SAHCP.html.

301. Thomas Bodenheimer, Kate Lorig, Halsted Holman, and Kevin Grumbach, "Patient Self-Management of Chronic Disease in Primary Care," *JAMA*, 20 November 2002. "People with chronic conditions are the principal care-givers. Each day, patients decide what they are going to eat, whether they will exercise and to what extent they will consume prescribed medicines."

302. David M. Eddy, "Variations in Physician Practice: The Role of Uncertainty," *Health Affairs*, Summer 1984.

303. Marie Skelton, "Report: Patient Illiteracy Threatens Health Care," *USA Today*, 25 March 2007.

304. Jane Brody, "The Importance of Knowing What the Doctor Is Talking About," *New York Times*, 30 January 2007.

305. "Reading for Your Life," *Philadelphia Inquirer,* circa 07 January 1994.

306. Jane Brody, "The Importance of Knowing What the Doctor Is Talking About," *New York Times,* 30 January 2007.

307. "Ill Health and Illiteracy: A Highly Dangerous Team," *New York Times,* 06 December 1995.

308. Catherine Arnst, "No Need for a Spoonful of Sugar," *Business Week,* 05 March 2007.

309. "Many Seniors Report Not Talking to Docs About Rx Medications," *Commonwealth Fund,* 13 February 2007.

310. Jessica Hopfield, Robert M. Linden, and Bradley J. Tevelow, "Getting Patients to Take Their Medicine," *McKinsey Quarterly,* November 2006.

311. "Many Americans Disregard Doctors' Course of Treatment," *Wall Street Journal,* 15 March 2007.

312. Tara Parker-Pope, "Testing Mistakes at the Family Doctor," *New York Times,* 14 Aug 2008.

313. This calculation is 0.95 to the twelfth power. In other words, it is a string of 12 instances of 0.95 multiplied together.

314. "Healthcare for Life," Medford Leas, downloaded 17 August 2009. See http://www.medfordleas.org/healthcare.htm.

315. "W. Edwards Deming," Wikipedia, http://en.wikipedia.org/wiki/W._Edwards_Deming, downloaded 07 Dec 2009.

316. Ibid.

317. One version of this fable can be found at http://aesopfables.com/cgi/aseop1.cgi?2&TheHareandtheTortoise.

318. The hare's contempt for the tortoise is a feature of some versions of the fable. See, for example, http://aesopfables.com/cgi/aesop1.cgi?2&TheHareandtheTortoise2&&haretort2.ram.

319. For a discussion of process management in hospitals, see David Leonhardt, "Making Health Care Better," *New York Times,* 08 November 2009.

320. Donald M. Berwick, "Continuous Improvement as an Ideal in Health Care," *New England Journal of Medicine,* 05 January 1989.

Chapter Twelve: Purpose

321. Sharon Sung, "Direct Reporting of Laboratory Test Results to Patients by Mail to Enhance Patient Safety," *Journal of General Internal Medicine,* October 2006.

322. Ibid.

323. Incidentally, this second solution would also solve the doctors' time problem.

324. Noel Gardner, conversation with the author, May 2008. Dr. Gardner has been involved in education of medical students for decades and noted that virtually all students reply with this answer when asked what their job is.

325. U.S. Department of Health and Human Services, Centers for Disease Control and Prevention, National Center for Health Statistics, "Health, United States, 2008," November 2008. The first two statistics come from Table 94 and the third from Table 106. All refer to data from the year 2006.

326. Many people would say that a "customer" is someone who writes the check (so to speak) to buy something. They would conclude that therefore the customer of health care is the government, which pays about half the tab in the United States, and employers, who pay another 25- 40%, depending on how you count. For the purpose of this chapter, customer is defined a bit differently. Health care can change or end people's lives. They have to live in the bodies treated. They also have to take many of the actions required to prevent or treat medical problems. For these reasons, I suggest that they should be viewed as the primary customers of health care.

327. Gina Kolata, "Cancer Group Has Concerns On Screenings," *New York Times*, 21 October 2009.

See also Gina Kolata, "New Guidelines Suggest Fewer Mammograms," *New York Times*, 17 November 2009. The subtitle reads "Reversal on Screening," and the article notes, "While many women do not think a screening test can be harmful, medical experts say the risks are real. A test can trigger unnecessary further tests, like biopsies, that can create extreme anxiety. And mammograms can find cancers that grow so slowly that they never would be noticed in a woman's lifetime, resulting in unnecessary treatment . . . One cancer death is prevented for every 1,904 women age 40 to 49 who are screened for 10 years."

328. Gina Kolata, "Cancer Group Has Concerns On Screenings," *New York Times*, 21 October 2009.

329. Gina Kolata, "Prostate Test Found to Save Few Lives," *New York Times*, 19 March 2009.

330. Ibid.

331. Ibid. The quotation is not a quotation from the article; it captures the data the article provides.

332. Tara Parker-Pope, "Screen or Not? What Those Prostate Studies Mean," *New York Times*, 24 March 2009, quoting Dr. Otis Brawley.

333. John Carey, "Do Cholesterol Drugs Do Any Good?" *Business Week*, 17 January 2008.

See also Tara Parker-Pope, "A Call for Caution in the Rush to Statins," *New York Times*, 18 November 2008.

334. Donald M. Berwick, "What 'Patient-Centered' Should Mean: Confessions of an Extremist," *Health Affairs* online, 19 May 2009.

335. Following are eight references spanning 15 years to support this impression:

From Lucian Leape, "Error in Medicine," *JAMA*, 21 December 1994: "Autopsy studies have shown high rates (35% to 40%) of missed diagnoses causing death."

From Lawrence K. Altman, "Diagnoses and the Autopsies Are Found to Differ Greatly," *New York Times*, 14 October 1998: "A new study has found a substantial discrepancy between the number of cancers detected during life and those found in autopsies. Despite advances in medical technology, the disparity between the diagnosis of cancer before and after death was 44 percent, similar to that found in studies conducted in earlier decades, said the authors."

From Atul Gawande, *Complications: A Surgeon's Notes on an Imperfect Science*, New York: Henry Holt, 2002, p. 197 of the paperback version, with footnotes on p. 262: "How often do autopsies turn up a major misdiagnosis in the cause of death? . . . According to three studies done in 1998 and 1999 . . . the figure is about 40 percent. A large review of autopsy studies concluded that in about a third of the misdiagnoses the patients would have been expected to live if proper treatment had been administered. . . . The most surprising fact of all: the rates at which misdiagnosis is detected in autopsy studies have not improved since at least 1938."

From Anahad O'Connor, "Deaths Go Unexamined and the Living Pay the Price," *New York Times*, 02 March 2004: "A growing number of missed or mistaken diagnoses are going unchecked, depriving doctors of a learning tool. And studies, including one published last week, find that autopsies uncover missed or incorrect diagnoses in up to 25 percent of hospital deaths."

From David Leonhardt, "Why Doctors So Often Get It Wrong," *New York Times*, 22 February 2006: "Studies of autopsies have shown that doctors seriously misdiagnose fatal illnesses about 20 percent of the time. So millions of patients are being treated for the wrong disease."

From "Because the Doctor Isn't Always Right," *CBS News*, May 07, 2006: "Experts find a 40 percent misdiagnosis rate."

From *Kaiser Daily Health Policy Report*, 29 November 2006: "The *Wall Street Journal* on Wednesday examined how Kaiser Permanente and the Department of Veterans Affairs 'are leading new efforts to improve diagnostic accuracy.' According to the *Journal*, 'diagnostic errors are the Achilles' heel of medicine — yet little has been done to prevent their deadly toll.' Studies have found that diagnostic errors occur in 10% to 30% of cases and 'generally stem from flaws in doctors' thinking, glitches in the health care system or some combination of both,' the *Journal* reports. According to a 2002 study conducted by the Agency for Healthcare Research and Quality, diagnostic errors that might have changed patient outcomes are found in 5% to 10% of all autopsies."

From "Alternative Diagnosis," www.wrongdiagnosis.com, downloaded 23 April 2009: "Misdiagnosis can and does occur and is reasonably common with error rates ranging from 1.4% in cancer biopsies to a high 20-40% misdiagnosis rate in emergency or ICU care. Surveys of patients also indicate the chance of experiencing a misdiagnosis to range from 8% to 40%."

336. Laura Landro, "Preventing the Tragedy of Misdiagnosis," *Wall Street Journal*, 29 November 2006.

337. Cathryn Gunther, health care strategist, in a conversation with the author, 03 December 2009, noted that it can be very difficult to arrive at a diagnosis. At the same time, doctors feel pressured to specify a diagnostic code — write down a diagnosis when filing an insurance claim — in order to support the need for certain tests, get paid for the consultation, etc. As a result, they go on record with a diagnosis — indicating a degree of certainty that they may not feel.

338. As an example, consider the story discussed in Chapter Five of the woman who was prescribed a diabetes drug for *five years* despite the fact that it caused a 70-pound weight gain. Other alternatives were readily available that did not have this side effect. Drawn from Mary Duenwald, "Is Your Medicine Cabinet Making You Fat?" *New York Times*, 16 August 2005.

339. John Carey, "Medical Guesswork," *Business Week,* 29 May 2006.

340. Ibid.

341. There are dozens, if not more, variations on SMART goals. This one is drawn from The Open Group and can be found at http://www.opengroup.org/architecture/togaf8-doc/arch/chap34.html#tag_35_09.

342. "1,001 Joint Replacement Patients Tell You What Doctors Can't," *Consumer Reports*, June 2006.

343. Robert Galvin, "A Deficiency of Will and Ambition': A Conversation with Donald Berwick," *Health Affairs*, 12 January 2005.

Chapter Thirteen: The Blind Men and the Elephant

344. One version of this story appears at http://www.geocities.com/Tokyo/Courtyard/1652/Elephant.html. Another version, with six blind men, appears at http://www.milk.com/random-humor/elephant_fable.html. The version in this book is an amalgam of the two.

345. Consider the perspective in "Health Care's Infectious Losses," by Paul O'Neill, *New York Times*, 06 July 2009: "Which of the [health reform] proposals will eliminate the annual toll of 300 million medication errors? . . . Which of the proposals will capture even a fraction of the roughly $1 trillion of annual 'waste' that is associated with the kinds of process failures [questions like this] imply? So far, the answer . . . is 'none.'"

Additionally, there is limited research indicating that many of these solutions actually move the dial. For example, see Sumit R. Majumdar and Stephen B. Soumerai, "The Unhealthy State of Health Policy Research," *Health Affairs*, 11 August 2009 (online). This article describes the flawed research that creates unsupported claims that Health Information Technology, Pay for Performance, and increased cost-sharing (Consumer-Directed Health Plans) yield improved results.

See also "Study Questions Effectiveness of Pay-for-Performance System," *Kaiser Daily Health Policy Report*, 10 March 2009.

346. "America's Uninsured Crisis: Consequences for Health and Health Care," Institute of Medicine, February 2009.

347. See, for example, Elizabeth Docteur and Robert A. Berenson, "How Does the Quality of U.S. Health Care Compare Internationally?" Robert Wood Johnson Foundation, August 2009, which notes, "If reform accomplishes no more than extending insurance coverage to the more than 45 million Americans without insurance, it will be an important step forward, but more is needed to ensure health care quality improvement."

See also Arnold Milstein, "Toxic Waste in the U.S. Health System," *Health Affairs Blog*, 02 June 2008, which notes that 24,000 people a year were expected to die as a result of lack of insurance. Contrast this number with the numbers of deaths from medical errors, from hospital acquired infections, and from other care-related problems noted in Chapter One.

348. Uwe Reinhardt, "Why Does U.S. Health Care Cost So Much? (Part II: Indefensible Administrative Costs)," *New York Times*, 21 November 2008. The article quotes a McKinsey study from 2003, which he extrapolates to 2008, estimating the excess spending (roughly, spending beyond what should be necessary to do the job) on administration to be $150 billion in 2008. McKinsey estimated that 85% of the excess spending on administration is related to the private insurance system. Thus, $150 billion x .85 = roughly $128 billion. Other researchers come up with even bigger numbers, but this one is big enough to make the point.

349. Gardiner Harris, "Prosecutors Plan Crackdown on Doctors Who Accept Kickbacks," *New York Times*, 04 March 2009.

350. Robert Pear, "Obama Push to Cut Health Costs Faces Tough Odds," *New York Times*, 12 May 2009. "Such cost-control devices have proved spectacularly ineffective in limiting the growth of Medicare spending on doctors' services."

351. "Birth Control Prices Soar on Campus," *MSNBC*, 23 March 2007.

352. "Decrease Price . . . Increase Supply?" *Healthcare Economist*, 27 October 2006. "When Medicare decides to reduce its fees, the quantity of medical services supplied by physicians actually increases."

353. Andrew Pollack, "The Minimal Impact of a Big Hypertension Study," *New York Times*, 28 November 2008.

354. Tara Parker-Pope, "A Hurdle for Health Reform: Patients and Their Doctors," *New York Times*, 03 March 2009.

See also Gardiner Harris, "Document Details Plan to Promote Costly Drug," *New York Times*, 02 September 2009, which starts off, "The pharmaceutical industry has developed thousands of medicines that have saved millions of lives, but it has also used its marketing muscle to successfully peddle expensive pills that are no more effective than older drugs sold at a fraction of the cost."

355. "Fewer Patients Using Health Care Provider Quality Ratings Web Sites to Make Decisions," *Kaiser Daily Health Policy Report*, 02 December 2008.

See also "2008 Update on Consumers' Views of Patient Safety and Quality Information," Kaiser Family Foundation, October 2008, which notes, "The share of the public now saying that they have seen and/or used information comparing the quality among various health care related providers has fallen back to levels last recorded in 2000. . . . Furthermore, people report real difficulty in finding comparative costs related [sic] information that many believe would help patients become more cost-conscious consumers of health care."

356. "Health Care Costs: A Primer — Key Information on Health Care Costs and Their Impact," Kaiser Family Foundation, August 2007.

357. Atul Gawande, "The Cost Conundrum," *New Yorker*, 01 June 2009, quoting a cardiac surgeon.

358. For a discussion of traditional quality measures in health care, see Anthony R. Kovner, *Health Care Delivery in the United States, Fourth Edition,* New York: Springer, 1990.

359. Regina Herzlinger, *Market-Driven Health Care: Who Wins, Who Loses In the Transformation of America's Largest Service Industry,* New York: Addison-Wesley, 1997.

360. Michael E. Porter and Elizabeth Olmsted Teisberg, *Redefining Health Care: Creating Value-Based Competition on Results,* Boston: Harvard Business School, 2006.

361. Consider, for example, the data reported by Siri Carpenter, "Treating an Illness Is One Thing. What About a Patient With Many?" *New York Times,* 31 March 2009. "Two-thirds of people over age 65, and almost three-quarters of people over 80, have multiple chronic health conditions, and 68 percent of Medicare spending goes to people who have five or more chronic diseases. . . . Yet people with multiple health problems . . . are largely overlooked both in medical research and in the nation's clinics and hospitals. The default position is to treat complicated patients as collections of malfunctioning body parts rather than as whole human beings."

362. NCQA (The National Committee for Quality Assurance) has published an impressive 32-page document, "Physician Practice Connections-Patient Centered Medical Home Companion Guide," available at http://www.ncqa.org/tabid/1034/Default.aspx. It details the standards a medical practice must meet to garner recognition as a medical home.

363. Ibid.

Chapter Fourteen: The Path Forward

364. Roni Caryn Rabin, "Bad Habits Asserting Themselves," *New York Times,* 09 June 2009. The percentage of people age 40-74 who:

- Eat five fruits and vegetables a day: 26%
- Don't smoke: 84%
- Exercised 30 minutes 3x week   43%

Multiplying these together yields the conclusion that 9.4% of people did all three.

Then, from the "Health Behaviors of Adults: United States 2002-2004," U.S. Department of Health and Human Services, Centers for Disease Control and Prevention, National Center for Health Statistics, Vital and Health Statistics, Series 10, Number 230, September 2006, it develops that 61% of the population drinks (Table 3.1) and 20% of them have had more than five drinks in a single day in the last year (Table 3.3.) This means that, understating the case somewhat, .61 x .20 = 12% of the population might be considered problem drinkers, yielding 88% who are not. Factoring this in to the calculation above, about 8% of the population is doing well on all four measures.

See also Dana E. King, Arch G. Mainous III, Mark Carnemolla, and Charles J. Everett, "Adherence to Healthy Lifestyle Habits in US Adults, 1988-2006," *American Journal of Medicine,* June 2009. It paints a bleaker picture: "Only 3% of US adults adhered to 4 healthy lifestyle characteristics (5 fruits and vegetables a day, regular physical activity, maintaining a healthy weight, and not smoking)."

365. Chris Browne, "Hagar the Horrible," *Daily Courier,* 27 February 2009.

366. Assume 37 million hospital stays averaging 6 days each, per "Health, United States, 2008," U.S. Department of Health and Human Services, Centers for Disease Control and Prevention, National Center for Health Statistics, 2009, Table 106. Further assume that each individual is visited 10 times a day by various doctors, nurses, aides, and other people providing care or support. That's 37,000,000 stays x 6 days x 10 interactions with care providers = 2,220,000,000 opportunities to pass on an infection. (That's 2.2 billion.)

According to the CDC, 1.7 million people pick up infections in the hospital and 99,000 die. See "Estimates of Healthcare-Associated Infections," Centers for Disease Control and Prevention, 30 May 2007. One simplified way to look at the numbers is this: 1,700,000 of the 2,220,000,000 contacts resulted in transmission of a perceptible infection. That's 17 out of 22,200 contacts, or less than one in a thousand. And it means that infections that cause deaths are passed on to patients 99,000 times out of 2.2 billion encounters. That's one out of every 22,000 times.

(The number of 10 contacts was chosen somewhat arbitrarily and probably understates the number of contacts by quite a bit — just delivering and picking up meal trays would yield 6 contacts a day. The effect of lowballing the number of contacts is that it paints a worse picture than is accurate. Instead of one infection for every 22,000 encounters, it's probably more like one infection for every 50,000 encounters, or more. You are welcome to estimate a different number of contacts if you like and see what the result is.)

I can hear the statisticians objecting: if someone acquires an infection in her first encounter with a doctor on the first day of a hospital stay, you don't really know if more germs are transmitted in subsequent encounters; they get drowned out, so to speak. The point is that the percentage of people harmed by hospital-acquired infections is relatively small compared to the number of opportunities to cause harm.

367. "Wash Your Hands. No, *Really.*" *Prevention*, March 2009.

368. S. Jay Olshansky, Douglas J. Passaro, Ronald C. Hershow, Jennifer Layden, Bruce A. Carnes, Jacob Brody, Leonard Hayflick, Robert N. Butler, David B. Allison, and David S. Ludwig, "A Potential Decline in Life Expectancy in the United States in the 21st Century," *New England Journal of Medicine*, 17 March 2005.

See also the 2008 video at www.healthiestnation.org, which notes, "For the first time our children will have shorter life expectancies than ours."

369. This view is echoed in an article by David Leonhardt, "Fat Tax," *New York Times*, 16 August 2009. "The debate over health care reform has so far revolved around how insurers, drug companies, doctors, nurses and government technocrats might be persuaded to change their behavior. And for the sake of the economy and the federal budget, they do need to change their behavior. But there has been far less discussion about how the rest of us might also change our behavior. It's as if we have little responsibility for our own health. We instead outsource it to something called the health care system."

The article continues, "The promise of that system is undeniably alluring: whatever your ailment, a pill or a procedure will fix it. Yet the promise hasn't been kept. For all the miracles that modern medicine really does perform, it is not the primary determinant of most people's health. J. Michael McGinnis, a senior scholar at the Institute of Medicine, has estimated that only 10 percent of early deaths are the result of substandard medical care. About 20 percent stem from social and physical environments, and 30 percent from genetics. The biggest contributor, at 40 percent, is behavior." The article goes on to argue for a new public health effort aimed at supporting higher activity levels, better nutrition, and so forth.

370. Kenneth E. Thorpe, David H. Howard, and Katya Galactionova, "Differences in Disease Prevalence as a Source of the U.S.-European Health Care Spending Gap," *Health Affairs* online, 02 October 2007.

371. Matthew 7:3, New International Version (1984), downloaded from www.biblegateway.com on 03 Dec 2009.

372. "Health, United States, 2008," U.S. Department of Health and Human Services, Centers for Disease Control and Prevention, National Center for Health Statistics, 2009. Table 108 notes that "all employed civilians" in 2007 total 146,047,000. Health care employment for 2007 was 14,687,000 people.

See also Gerald F. Seib, "U.S. Psyche Bedevils Health Effort," *Wall Street Journal*, 04 August 2009, which notes that not only are there more than 14 million jobs in health care today, but it's expected to add "a staggering three million new wage and salaried jobs in the next decade or so, more than any other industry."

373. "Health Care Spending Will Account for One-Fifth of GDP in 2018, Federal Government Will Pay More Than 50% of Those Costs, According to CMS Report," *Kaiser Daily Health Policy Report*, 24 February 2009.

374. Micah Hartman, Anne Martin, Patricia McDonnell, Aaron Catlin, and the National Health Expenditure Accounts Team, "National Health Spending In 2007: Slower Drug Spending Contributes to Lowest Rate of Overall Growth Since 1998," *Health Affairs*, January/February 2009.

375. Paul Otellini, "Making Health Care Personal," *Politico*, 27 July 2009. The author is CEO of Intel Corp.

376. Ibid.

377. "Constant Stress Linked to Overeating," *United Press International*, 14 May 2008.

See also "Why We Overeat and Overspend," *The Week*, 13 June 2009. This research showed that people overeat and overspend when they have been thinking about death. The idea for the research arose as a result of data showing that sales of "indulgent snacks" skyrocketed after the 9/11 terrorist attacks. While this study is focused on just one cause of stress, thinking about death, it seems plausible to suggest that many causes of stress might result in similar behavior. The data on overeating certainly suggest such a conclusion.

378. "Constant Stress Linked to Overeating," *United Press International*, 14 May 2008.

379. Edward T. Creagan, "How Do I Control Stress-Induced Weight Gain?" *MayoClinic.com*, 17 August 2009, found at http://www.mayoclinic.com/health/stress/an01128.

380. "Stress Symptoms: Effects on Your Body, Feelings and Behavior," *MayoClinic.com*, 20 February 2009, found at http://www.mayoclinic.com/health/stress-ymptoms/SR00008_D.

381. Rob Stein, "Baby Boomers Appear To Be Less Healthy Than Parents," *Washington Post*, 20 April 2007.

382. Ibid.

383. Kathleen Fackelmann, "Stress Can Ravage the Body, Unless the Mind Says No," *USA Today*, 22 March 2005.

384. Ron French, "Losing the Battle of the Bulge," *Detroit News*, 27 September 2006.

385. Nothing contained herein should be construed as personalized medical advice.

386. Stephanie Winston, *Getting Out From Under: Redefining Your Priorities in an Overwhelming World*, Reading: Perseus, 1999.

Another resource for people seeking to understand how to make different choices is Gerald Corey & Marianne Schneider Corey's *I Never Knew I Had a Choice*, now in its 9th edition (Monterey: Brooks/Cole, 2008.)

387. M. P. Dunleavey, "It Might Pay to Follow Your Bliss," *New York Times*, 16 June 2007.

388. Anthony Shih, Karen Davis, Stephen Schoenbaum, Anne Gauthier, Rachel Nuzum, and Douglas McCarthy, *Organizing the U.S. Health Care Delivery System for High Performance*, ed. Martha Hostetter, The Commonwealth Fund, 7 August 2008.

Chapter Fifteen: Surviving the Geeks-in-Garages Era

389. http://www.washingtonpavilion.org/VisualArtsCenter/events/ punchcardart.cfm.

390. The IBM Archives (at www.ibm.com) provide a sense of the magnitude of the change from centralized computing (data centers and mainframes) to decentralized (widespread use of personal computers in addition to mainframes): "It wasn't that long before the August 1981 debut of the IBM PC that an IBM computer often cost as much as $9 million and required an air-conditioned quarter-acre of space and 60 people to run and keep it loaded with instructions. The IBM PC changed all that. It was a very small machine that could . . . process information faster than those ponderous mainframes of the 1960s . . . for a price tag of less than $1,600." Now imagine a similar revolution in health care, from centralized activity run by experts to decentralized activity handled by individuals using systems created by experts.

391. H. Gilbert Welch, "To Overhaul the System, 'Health' Needs Redefining," *New York Times*, 28 July 2009.

392. Michael Blastland and Andrew Dilnot, "When Numbers Deceive," *The Week*, 27 February 2009, an extract from their book, *The Numbers Game*. The entire example described here is drawn from their work.

393. Ibid.

394. Jerome Groopman, *How Doctors Think*, Boston: Houghton Mifflin, 2008.

395. Melinda Beck, "Bedside Manner: Advocating for a Relative in the Hospital," *Wall Street Journal*, 28 October 2008.

396. See, for example, the "Medicare Part D Medication Therapy Management (MTM) Programs 2008 Fact Sheet," found at http://www.cms.hhs.gov/PrescriptionDrugCovContra/Downloads/MTMFactSheet.pdf.

397. Steve Sternberg and Jack Gillum, "'Double Failure' at USA's Hospitals," *USA Today*, 10 July 2009.

398. Jared A. Favole, "Readmitted Patients Cost Billions," *Wall Street Journal*, 01 April 2009.

399. Ibid.

400. Reed Abelson, "In Health Care, Cost Isn't Proof of High Quality," *New York Times*, 14 Jun 2007. The article notes: "The fact that there is no connection between quality and cost is one of the dirty secrets of medicine."

Consider also Laura Yasaitis, Elliott S. Fisher, Jonathan S. Skinner, and Amitabh Chandra, "Hospital Quality and Intensity of Spending: Is There an Association?" *Health Affairs*, 21 May 2009, which states flatly, "Hospitals' performance on quality of care is not associated with the intensity of their spending," meaning that there's no connection between the cost and the quality of care the patient gets.

401. Alex Berenson, "Weighing the Costs of a CT Scan's Look Inside the Heart," *New York Times*, 29 June 2008.

402. Andrew Pollack, "The Minimal Impact of a Big Hypertension Study," *New York Times*, 28 November 2008.

See also Richard A. Friedman, "New Drugs Have Allure, Not Track Record," *New York Times*, 19 May 2009. This article describes a failure to offer "the single most effective treatment" because it was an old drug.

403. Ceci Connolly, "U.S. 'Not Getting What We Pay For,'" *Washington Post*, 30 November 2008. The quotation is attributed to Gary Kaplan, who runs Virginia Mason Medical Center in Seattle, widely reputed to be one of the best hospital/clinic organizations in the country.

404. M. Laurant, D. Reeves, R. Hermens, J. Braspenning, R. Grol, and B. Sibbald, "Substitution of Doctors by Nurses in Primary Care," Cochrane Collaboration, 20 April 2005, found at http://www.cochrane.org/reviews/en/ab001271.html.

405. S. Horrocks, E. Anderson, and C. Salisbury, "Systematic Review of Whether Nurse Practitioners Working in Primary Care Can Provide Equivalent Care to Doctors," *BMJ*, 06 April 2002.

Chapter Sixteen: Chaos

406. Chris Koyanagi, Sandra Forquer, and Elaine Alfano, "Medicaid Policies To Contain Psychiatric Drug Costs," *Health Affairs*, March/April 2005.

407. Ibid.

408. Janet Adamy, "Doctors Fight Penalty for Heavy Drug Use," *Wall Street Journal*, 02 October 2009.

409. Ibid.

410. "Taxation on Tobacco," *Encyclopedia of Public Health*, found at http://www.enotes.com/public-health-encyclopedia/taxation-tobacco.

411. "One Year after State Cigarette Tax Increase, Smoking at Lowest Rate Ever Recorded," *Press Release*, New York State Department of Health, 04 June 2009. To clarify, this doesn't mean that the percent of people who smoked used to be 16.7% + the 12% reduction in smokers = 28.7% who used to smoke. It means that about 19% of the people used to smoke. 12% of 19% (that is, .12 x .19) = 2.3%. So the new percentage of smokers is 19% - 2.3% = 16.7%.

412. "More Tax Hike Ideas," *Kiplinger Tax Letter*, 29 May 2009.

413. Elizabeth Lopatto, "Artificial Sweetener Linked to Weight Gain, Scientists Say," *Bloomberg*, 10 February 2008.

See also Melinda Beck, "Why That Big Meal You Just Ate Made You Hungry," *Wall Street Journal*, 14 April 2009. It reports on a book by Louis J. Aronne titled *The Skinny*.

414. Elizabeth Lopatto, "Artificial Sweetener Linked to Weight Gain, Scientists Say," *Bloomberg*, 10 February 2008.

415. Melinda Beck, "Why That Big Meal You Just Ate Made You Hungry," *Wall Street Journal*, 14 April 2009.

416. Ibid.

417. Michelle Andrews, "If Your Waistline Grows, Should Your Premiums, Too?" *New York Times*, 08 October 2009.

418. The math works like this: Suppose your health insurance costs $1,000 (a round number to make the math easy). A 50% discount would mean you might pay as little as $500. If you don't qualify for the discount and other people in your workplace do, they'd be paying $500 and you'd be paying $1,000 — twice as much as they are.

419. Steven A. Schroeder, "We Can Do Better – Improving the Health of the American People," *New England Journal of Medicine*, 20 September 2007.

420. "UnitedHealth: Stick to Your Meds, Get $20 Off Next Prescription," *Wall Street Journal*, 28 August 2009.

421. Marelisa Fabrega, "The Future Belongs to Those Who Are Intrinsically Motivated," *Stanford Wellsphere*, 02 September 2009, found at http://stanford.wellsphere.com/stress-relief-article/the-future-belongs-to-those-who-are-intrinsically-motivated/787624.

422. Ibid.

423. Alfie Kohn, "Group Grade Grubbing versus Cooperative *Learning*," *Educational Leadership*, February 1991.

See also Marelisa Fabrega, "The Future Belongs to Those Who Are Intrinsically Motivated," *Stanford*

Wellsphere, http://stanford.wellsphere.com/stress-relief-article/the-future-belongs-to-those-who-are-intrinsically-motivated/787624, 02 September 2009.

424. John Tauer, "Latrell Sprewell + Pizza Hut < Intrinsic Motivation," *Psychology Today*, 30 June 2009.

425. Melissa Melayna, "Impacts of Extrinsic Motivation Techniques on Intrinsic Motivation," *Associated Content*, 28 June 2007.

426. Ibid.

427. "CMS Improves Patient Safety for Medicare and Medicaid by Addressing Never Events," *Press Release*, U.S. Department of Health and Human Services, Centers for Medicare & Medicaid Services, 04 August 2008.

428. Andrew Pollack, "Drug Deals Tie Prices to How Well Patients Do," *New York Times*, 23 April 2009.

429. Jeffrey Kluger, "Drive-Thru Medical: Retail Health Clinics' Good Marks," *Time*, 01 September 2009.

430. Catherine M. DesRoches, "Electronic Health Records in Ambulatory Care — A National Survey of Physicians," *New England Journal of Medicine*, 03 July 2008. About 17% of doctors use electronic medical records.

In contrast, see the Convenient Care Association's quality standards, at http://www.ccaclinics.org/index.php?option=com_content&view=article&id=6&Itemid=13. The Convenient Care Association is the trade association for retail clinics. One of the requirements for membership in the Convenient Care Association is to "use Electronic Health Records (EHR) to ensure high-quality efficient care. All CCA Members are committed to providing all patients with the opportunity to share health information with other providers electronically or in paper format."

431. Lynn Lofton, "Medical Clinics Inside Retail Stores Opening in State," *Mississippi Business Journal*, 11 December 2006.

432. Jeffrey Kluger, "Drive-Thru Medical: Retail Health Clinics' Good Marks," *Time*, 01 September 2009.

433. "Retail Medical Clinics Can Provide Care at Lower Cost, Similar Quality as Other Medical Settings," *Press Release*, Rand Corporation, 31 August 2009. This press release announces the results of an independent study of retail clinics, published in the *Annals of Internal Medicine*, 01 September 2009. "The RAND study found no evidence to support the concerns."

434. Paul H. Keckley and Howard R. Underwood, "Medical Tourism: Update and Implications," Deloitte Center for Health Solutions, 23 October 2009.

435. Christopher J. Gearon, "Get a Hip Replaced and See the World," *Kiplinger's Retirement Report*, April 2008.

See also Walecia Konrad, "Going Abroad to Find Affordable Health Care," *New York Times*, 21 March 2009.

436. Paul H. Keckley and Howard R. Underwood, "Medical Tourism: Update and Implications," Deloitte Center for Health Solutions, 23 October 2009.

437. "Telemedicine and Telehealth," Centers for Medicare & Medicaid Services, http://www.cms.hhs.gov/Telemedicine, 15 September 2009.

438. Will Engle, "Home Telehealth," *telemedicine information exchange*, March 2009.

439. All of the information about group visits, unless otherwise noted, comes from Edward Noffsinger, "Using Group Visits Effectively in Chronic Illness Treatment Programs," a talk given at the Institute for Healthcare Improvement's 19th Annual National Forum on Quality Improvement in Health Care, 11

December 2007. Noffsinger has written a book, *Running Group Visits in Your Practice*, New York: Springer, 2009, which describes this topic in further detail.

440. Ibid.

441. Parija B. Kavilanz, "Doctors' Orders: Avoid Insurance," *CNNMoney.com*, 17 August 2009.

442. Melinda Beck, "Health Matters," *Wall Street Journal*, 14 February 2009.

443. Ibid.

444. Christopher J. Gearon, "Doctor House Calls in the Information Age," *Kiplinger's Retirement Report,* March 2009.

Consider also the experience of Kaiser-Permanente, which provides care for 8.5 million people. Doctors at Kaiser are paid a salary, rather than paid for each visit or procedure. The use of e-mail with patients is "a condition of employment," said Anna-Lisa Silvestre, "The Informed Patient: Reinventing the Patient-Provider Relationship (Virtually)," 5th Annual Consumer Health Care Congress, 01 October 2009.

445. Carleen Hawn, "Games for Health: The Latest Tool in the Medical Care Arsenal," *Health Affairs*, online 04 August 2009. The next three notes reference this article as well.

446. Ibid.

447. Ibid.

448. Ibid.

Chapter Seventeen: The Future When Health Care Is About You

449. Leila Abboud, "Drug Makers Seek to Bar 'Placebo Responders' From Trials," *Wall Street Journal*, 18 June 2004.

450. "Farewell to Scientist Who Discovered Penicillin," *BBC*, 11 March 1955, found at http://news.bbc.co.uk/onthisday/hi/dates/stories/march/11/newsid_2538000/2538043.stm.

451. "Alexander Fleming," Wikipedia, http://en.wikipedia.org/wiki/Alexander_Fleming, 06 December 2009.

452. Sharon Begley, "Why Thinking You Got a Workout May Make Your Body Healthier," *Wall Street Journal*, 02 February 2007.

453. "Unnecessary Operations," *Prevention*, 07 July 2007.

See also "Comparative Effectiveness: Back Surgery Remains Popular Despite Poor Study Results," *Kaiser Daily Health Policy Report*, 24 August 2009, which quotes two studies reported on in the *New England Journal of Medicine* which concluded that one type of back surgery is "no more effective than a sham surgery."

454. Nicholas Bakalar, "Reminder to Smokers: Your Lungs Are Aging," *New York Times*, 11 March 2008.

455. Ibid.

456. Jacob Goldstein, "MacArthur Genius Award: Reducing Falls in the Elderly," *Wall Street Journal*, 22 September 2009.

457. Ibid.

458. Siri Carpenter, "Treating an Illness is One Thing. What About a Patient with Many?" *New York Times*, 31 March 2009.

459. Ibid.

460. "The Public Needs to Understand the Uncertainty of Medicines Regulation," *Scrip*, 23 January 2006. As quoted in Chapter Six, "Healthcare systems have always transferred uncertainty and risk to the

patient. Managers, doctors and nurses are in control; they have certainty, it is the patient who usually does not know what is going to happen, or when or why. The risk is taken by the patient rather than the doctor."

461. "ED [Emergency Department] Patients More Satisfied If They Know Wait Times," *FierceHealthcare*, 31 July 2008.

462. Charles Adler, a doctor at the Mayo Clinic in Arizona, consultation, 03 June 2009.

463. The Mayo Clinic hasn't reached this point by accident. They put a great deal of effort into research to improve the experience of people treated there. See for example Barbara R. Spurrier's presentation in the session, "Signature Innovations to Transform the Delivery and Experience of Health Care," 6th Annual World Health Care Congress, 15 April 2009. Spurrier is Senior Administrator, Center for Innovation, Mayo Clinic.

464. Jordan Dolin, "Health Care's Greatest Untapped Resource: Patients," *chicagotribune.com*, 15 November 2009.

465. Leonard Cassuto, "John Madden Made Us Smarter," *Wall Street Journal*, 20 April 2009.

466. Ibid.

467. See a description of hyponatremia at http://www.mayoclinic.com/health/hyponatremia/DS00974.

468. Natasha Singer, "A Push to Spell Out a Drug's Risks and Benefits," *New York Times*, 26 February 2009.

469. Susan Edgman-Levitan, "NQF 2008 Implementation Conference on Care Coordination: Communications," The John D. Stoeckle Center for Primary Care Innovation, March 2008.

470. Laura Landro, "Weighty Choices, in Patients' Hands," *Wall Street Journal*, 04 August 2009.

See also John Carey, "Smarter Patients, Cheaper Care?" *Business Week*, 22 June 2009. The article is subtitled, "Better-informed medical decisions could cut billions in health-care costs as patients opt for cheaper treatments."

Separately, note that a mandate to include people in deciding what is going to be done to them is appropriate for patients who are mentally competent. That is, there are exceptions to the rule. However, today, there is no rule or expectation that most people will have a say in their treatment.

471. Richard M. Hoffman, Mick P. Couper, Brian J. Zikmund-Fisher, Carrie A. Levin, Mary McNaughton-Collins, Deborah L. Helitzer, John VanHoewyk, and Michael J. Barry, "Prostate Cancer Screening Decisions," *Archives of Internal Medicine*, 28 September 2009. In this case, "Health care providers emphasized the pros of testing in 71.4% of discussions but infrequently addressed the cons (32.0%)." This kind of disparity is common across testing and treatment discussions for many conditions.

472. Michael K. Paasche-Orlow, Holly A. Taylor, and Frederick L. Brancati, "Readability Standards for Informed-Consent Forms as Compared with Actual Readability," *New England Journal of Medicine*, 20 February 2003, which notes, "Almost half of Americans read at or below the 8th-grade level." The article goes on to suggest the use of materials written at a 4th-grade level.

See also Nancy Cotugna, Connie E. Vickery, and Kara M. Carpenter-Haefele, "Evaluation of Literacy Level of Patient Education Pages in Health-Related Journals," *Journal of Community Health*, June 2005.

See also "'What Did the Doctor Say?:' Improving Health Literacy to Protect Patient Safety," *Joint Commission*, 2007.

See also Mark Kutner, Elizabeth Greenberg, Ying Jin, and Christine Paulsen, "The Health Literacy of America's Adults: Results from the 2003 National Assessment of Adult Literacy," project officer Sheida White, National Center for Education Statistics, U.S. Department of Education, September 2006.

473. Donald M. Berwick, "What 'Patient-Centered' Should Mean: Confessions of An Extremist," *Health Affairs* online, 19 May 2009.

474. This is a complicated topic. I am not recommending eliminating step therapy, in which drugs that generally work and are less expensive are tried first, with a move toward more expensive or riskier drugs only if the first ones don't work. What I am suggesting is that instead of reaching a point where treatment is denied, less common but plausible treatment is authorized with the requirement that it be evaluated via a feedback loop at an appropriate interval. For some drugs, this might be two weeks. For others, it might be three months. Continuation of the drug would then be approved only if the feedback loop showed that the benefits exceeded the downsides.

In addition, what I am suggesting is that a feedback loop be created every time an individual is prescribed a drug for a chronic condition. Having a formal process to check for side effects and weigh benefits against the problems the drug may be causing could help people get treatments that work better for them much more frequently than is the case today. It could also help avoid some of the 8-10 million hospitalizations/year for adverse drug events. (See Chapter One.)

475. Cathryn Gunther, health care strategist, e-mail to the author, 12 May 2008.

476. Others also note the need to update medical education in order to improve how health care works. See Jacob Goldstein, "What Medical Education Has to Do With Health Reform," *Wall Street Journal*, 16 June 2009. He describes a report published by MedPac, which advises Congress on Medicare: "Specifically, the report cited 'the relative lack of formal training and experience in multidisciplinary teamwork, cost awareness in clinical decision making, comprehensive health information technology, and patient care in ambulatory [non-hospital] settings.' More generally, the report noted, medical residencies are largely based in hospitals." The full report — nearly 300 pages — is titled "Report to the Congress: Improving Incentives in the Medicare Program," and can be found at http://www.medpac.gov/documents/Jun09_EntireReport.pdf.

477. Siri Carpenter, "Treating an Illness is One Thing. What About a Patient with Many?" *New York Times*, 31 March 2009. "Two-thirds of people over age 65, and almost three-quarters of people over 80, have multiple chronic health conditions, and 68 percent of Medicare spending goes to people who have five or more chronic diseases . . . [but the] medical system [is] geared toward individual organs and diseases."

See also Siri Carpenter, "Is Your Parent Over-Medicated?" *Prevention*, December 2008.

478. Rosanne M. Leipzig, "The Patients Doctors Don't Know," *New York* Times, 02 July 2009.

479. Dennis McCullough, *My Mother, Your Mother: Embracing "Slow Medicine," the Compassionate Approach to Caring for Your Aging Loved One*, New York: Harper, 2008.

480. Consider, for example, Richard Friedman, "When All Else Fails, Blaming the Patient Often Comes Next," *New York Times*, 21 October 2008.

481. The logic of using people with less training but more focus on coaching the patient as the point of entry into health care first became evident to me in discussions with Kathy Beaudoin and Jeff Neely, health care strategists.

See also Alan Portner, "Doctor Shortage May Be Mitigated by Nurse Practitioners and Physician Assistants," *DC Public Policy Examiner*, 27 August 2009.

482. "Doctor Shortage and Disparities After Reform Examined, Nurses Prepare for Changing Role," *Kaiser Daily Health Policy Report*, 03 August 2009.

483. Arthur Garson, "The Grandparents Corps: A New Primary Care Model," *Health Affairs* blog, 28 September 2009.

484. Ibid.

485. Alan Portner, "Doctor Shortage May Be Mitigated by Nurse Practitioners and Physician Assistants," *DC Public Policy Examiner*, 27 August 2009.

See also "Doctor Shortage and Disparities After Reform Examined, Nurses Prepare for Changing Role," *Kaiser Daily Health Policy Report*, 03 August 2009.

486. Anna-Lisa Silvestre, Kaiser Permanente, "The Informed Patient: Reinventing the Patient-Provider Relationship (Virtually)," 5th Annual Consumer Health Care Congress, 01 October 2009.

487. Ibid.

488. "Facebook," Wikipedia entry downloaded 08 November 2009.

489. "Twitter," Wikipedia entry, downloaded 10 November 2009.

490. "YouTube," Wikipedia entry, downloaded 08 November 2009.

491. "Second Life," Wikipedia entry, downloaded 08 November 2009.

492. "PatientsLikeMe," Wikipedia entry, downloaded 08 November 2009.

493. Phil Baumann, "140 Health Care Uses for Twitter," *phil baumann online*, 19 January 2009. The tagline for this site is "Health is social."

494. "Second Life's Health Care Options Praised," *Virtual Worlds News*, 29 May 2009, reporting on a University of Toronto research study, Leslie Beard, Kumanan Wilson, Dante Morra, and Jennifer Keelan, "A Survey of Health-Related Activities on Second Life," *Journal of Medical Internet Research*, 22 May 2009.

495. Benjamin Heywood, "Social Networks — The Power and Potential for Social Networks and Online Communities in Health Care," 5th Annual Consumer Health Care Congress, 01 October 2009.

496. Ibid.

497. Thomas Goetz, "Practicing Patients," *New York Times*, 23 March 2008.

INDEX

Please visit
www.killercure.net

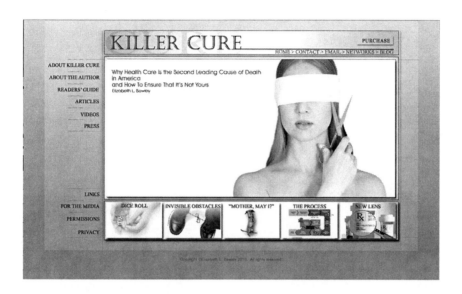

The website offers additional resources, such as:

- Printable version of the Readers' Discussion Guide
- Author's blog
- Author's videos

Coming in Autumn 2010:

- Workbook for *Killer Cure* to help you apply its thinking to your life
- Other resources to help you get what you need from health care

LaVergne, TN USA
17 May 2010
183002LV00003B/19/P